Intermittent Fasting

Built To Fast
Your True Intermittent Fasting Guide

By Emily Moore

TABLE OF CONTENTS

INTRODUCTION

Dieting is hard! There are so many options available, that sometimes it can feel *overwhelming* – you find yourself not even knowing where to begin. Or maybe you've tried them all – the gluten free diet, the Atkins diet, the Paleo diet – and *none* of them *have worked*, so you want to try something new.

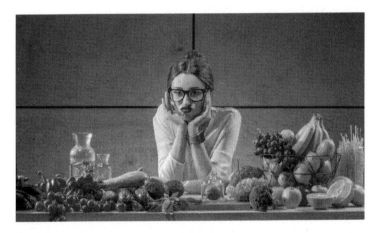

This is where **intermittent fasting** comes in. It's one of the hottest new ways to lose weight, and for very good reason! This isn't a diet; it's a *pattern of eating*. It's a way of **scheduling your meals so you get the most out of them.**

There are a great *number of benefits* to choosing this method, including:

- It's scientifically proven to help you **lose weight** and stomach fat.

- It can **improve your health** – helping with conditions such as diabetes and heart issues.

- It can also help **ward off diseases**, helping you in the long run.

- It's really good for your brain.

- It can actually help you **live longer**.

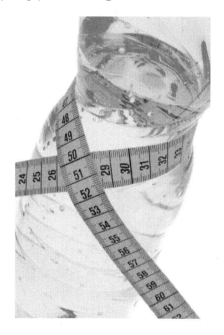

Of course, we will go into more detail of how intermittent fasting can help you turn around your life, during this book. In fact, you won't be able to find a more comprehensive guide on the market. Not only does it cover the *hottest diets to try*, it'll also ensure that you're fully equipped by giving you *tips to manage your fast*, while *keeping you safe* in the process.

On top of all of this, you will also be able to see a selection of *scientific studies* that have been conducted with regards to intermittent fasting – proving that the health, weight and brain benefits are genuine. Once you've had a look at exactly what has been researched for fasting, you'll be more convinced than ever. Whatever your end goal is – you'll see how **you can achieve it with fasting**.

Basically, it's everything you need, all in one place. By the time you have finished reading, you'll have everything you need to get you started with the **perfect intermittent fasting diet for you** –so don't put it off any longer, let's get started!

INTERMITTENT FASTING

What Is It?

Fasting is the process of abstaining from food and drink for a certain amount of time. **Intermittent fasting (IF)** involves a cycle of eating and fasting. It's so popular because it doesn't so much dictate *what* you should eat – thus eliminating lots of people who are on specialized diets, or don't enjoy certain foods – it's more based on *when* you should eat.

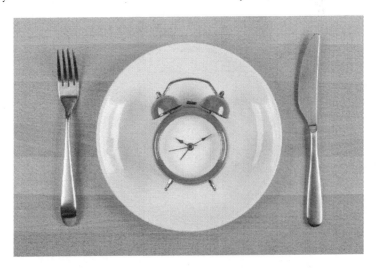

There are many different ways that you can do this fast – there is nothing set in stone about it, which means you can fit it into your lifestyle no matter what. We will look at some examples at how you can bring this into your life, and what sort of things you will want to eat to get the most out of your foods, later on in this book. As for now, let's have a look at *how* **intermittent fasting works.**

As already stated, **intermittent fasting *isn't* a diet**. It's a way of eating that humans have been doing for centuries. In the past, this may have been down to necessity – there just wasn't anything to eat available –being un-well, or religion. Many belief systems have periods of fasting, proving that it's doable, healthy and actually quite a natural way to feed.

In fact, there's a lot of evidence to demonstrate that 'starving' yourself for a little bit each day can have a **very positive impact on your health** – not just your weight. This is because it takes six to eight hours for your body to metabolize your glycogen stores and after that you start to burn fat. How-ever, if you are replenishing this glycogen by eating every eight hours or so, you make it far more difficult for your body to use your fat stores as fuel. Basically, you need to ensure that you give yourself a break from food to allow your body to do what needs to be done.

A Word About Metabolism

The way that our bodies lose or gain weight is primarily down to our **metabolism**. Simply put, this is the chemicals inside our bodies that convert food into energy. We need four main macronutrients to make this process happen:

- Proteins

- Fats

- Carbohydrates

- Nucleic Acids (found in DNA)

These factors can be found in food, and the **food pyramid** has been created to ensure that we're getting enough of these for our bodies to function properly.

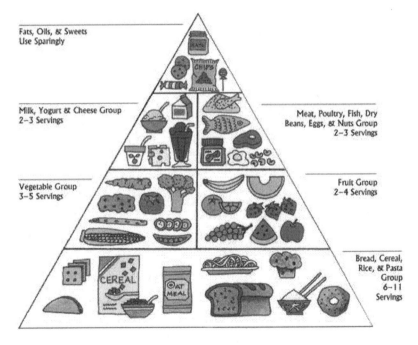

Our bodies then break down the things that we eat, and use them for energy. **The speed** that this is done determines how much weight we either gain or lose. This speed is affected by a great number of factors, including:

- *Age* – unfortunately, the older you get, the slower your metabolism becomes.

- *Body size* – if you're taller or heavier, your metabolism will need to work much harder to get the job done.

- *Muscle mass* – a higher muscle mass often leads to a more successful metabolism.

- *Gender* – men have a speedier metabolism than women.

- *Activity level* – exercise has a massive impact on the way that your metabolism works. The more you move, the better it will be.

- *Hormonal factors* – certain hormones and related illnesses will affect your metabolism.

- *Genetics* – you should be able to get a glimpse of how your metabolism will work from your family history.

- *Environmental factors* – the weather can actually impact on your metabolic rate. If it's very hot or cold, your system needs to work much harder for this process to work.

- *Diet* – eating healthily, only when you're hungry and at a scheduled time can make your metabolism work more effectively.

- *Drugs* – prescription drugs, caffeine and nicotine can slow down your metabolism.

As you can see from this list, the only factors that *you* have any control over is muscle mass and exercise – you can work out to improve this – and diet and drugs – what *you* chose to put into your body, will determine how it works and feels. **Fasting is extremely useful for speeding up your metabolism**, as shown by these points made:

- It eliminates waste from the body that have accumulated from normal eating and drinking. This gives your metabolism a boost.

- It activates the human growth hormone, which helps your body to burn fat and maintain muscle.

- It regulates digestion which promotes healthy bowel function and helps your metabolic rate to increase.

- It regulates blood sugar meaning that you don't feel ravenous.

- It improves your eating habits as you'll want to get the most out of your calorie limit. Healthy eating gives your metabolism the best chance at working at its optimum speed.

- Fasting actually slows the aging process, helping your metabolism to stay younger for longer.

So as you have seen, calorie restriction can help us lose weight and feel a lot healthier, but this is extremely challenging as *hunger is one of our primary drives*. Fortunately, studies have shown that intermittent fasting is a much easier way of achieving the same effect.

Health Benefits Of Fasting

Here is a list of **health benefits that fasting can help you achieve** – proving that it's about much more than just weight loss:

- Fasting **Improves Insulin Sensitivity** – this allows you to tolerate carbohydrates (sugar) better than if you didn't fast. A study showed that after periods of fasting, insulin becomes more effective in telling cells to take up glucose from blood.

- Fasting **Speeds Up The Metabolism** – your digestive system is given a rest, which energizes your metabolism.

- Fasting **Promotes Longevity** – studies have shown how the lifespan of people in certain cultures increased due to their diets.

- Fasting **Improves Hunger** – it actually takes between 12 to 24 hours to feel real hunger. You'll notice this as you fast.

- Fasting **Improves Your Brain Function** – this is because it boosts the production of a protein called *brain-derived neurotrophic factor* (BDNF.)

- Fasting **Improves Your Immune System** – this is because it reduces free radical damage, regulates inflammatory conditions in the body and starves off cancer cell formation. It's primal instinct to focus more on rest than food when you're sick.

- Fasting **Helps Clear The Skin And Prevent Acne** – this is because with the body temporarily freed from digestion, it's able to focus its regenerative energies on other systems.

Body Reactions To Fasting

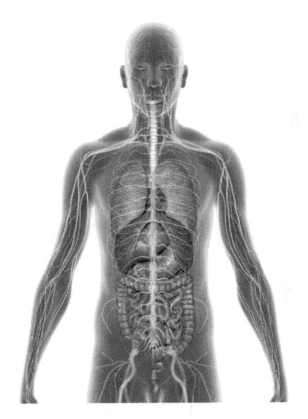

Here's what happens to your body during a fast:

1. Breakdown of body fat.

This is the part that leads to weight loss and helps reduce the risk of heart disease, strokes, cancer, diabetes, etc.

2. Cholesterol deposits break down.

Waste is quickly eliminated through a fast – and this includes cholesterol, which is normally stored within the lining of the blood vessels. The levels of cholesterol *can* actually go up within the first week of the fast as the body detoxifies, but it will soon decrease.

3. Fibrinolysis.

Dangerous blood clots that can build up within your body can be more easily broken down while on a fast. This process is known as fibrinolysis.

4. Accelerated autolysis.

Each cell in the body contains the seeds of its own destruction. When the need presents, itself, the cell will release its own self-destructive enzymes and self-destruct. This is autolysis. During the fast, the process of autolysis leads to the breakdown of this type of tissue which has hampered normal functioning.

5. Increased diuresis.

Diuresis is the excretion by the kidneys of salt and water. While fasting, the body spontaneously and automatically eliminates salt and water without damaging body tissues. This diuresis is of tremendous health benefit.

6. Accelerated phagocytosis.

While fasting, the ability of the body's defensive army of white blood cells to destroy virulent bacteria and digest waste material is accelerated. The white blood cells from the fasting person were significantly more effective at killing virulent bacteria.

4 Most Common Fasting Styles

Below is a guide to the **four most common fasting styles**. This list isn't extensive, it only covers the most popular, but it will certainly give you something to think about when it comes to your own goals and aims.

1. The Periodic Fast (Eat Stop Eat)

This is usually the 24 hour fast which you take periodically. This can be started at any time of the day and can be done once or twice weekly. This type of fast is also examined at great detail by **Brad Pilon** (*bradpilon.com*), where he recommends a 24 hour fast every 3-5 days for weight loss.

2. LeanGains

This method involves fasting for 16 hours at a time – for example, between 10pm until 2pm. After this, food is consumed in 3 meals during the remaining 8-hour window. LeanGains is written about by **Martin Berkhan** (*www.leangains.com*), who also includes details about exercise in this plan. So if you want to fast and continue working out, then this might be the plan for you.

3. The Warrior Diet

This fast is one step up from LeanGains. This method promotes just one single, healthy meal per day – typically dinner. A study conducted by Stote *et al (ajcn.nutrition.org/content/85/4/981.full)*. looks into this in more detail. In this study, participants of normal weight consumed adequate energy to maintain body weight in one meal per day or 3 meals per day for 8 weeks. Despite consumption of the same number of calories, participants lost weight during the 1 meal per day period vs. the 3 meal per day period. In fact, fat mass was significantly reduced and lean body mass tended to be greater after 8 weeks of 1 meal per day. However, hunger steadily increased during the 8-week study period with only 1 meal per day, suggesting that appetite hormones did not acclimate.

4. Alternate day fasting

This is more of an intermittent style of fasting. Food is consumed for 24 hours, then restricted for the next day. Heilbronn *et al.* (*www.ncbi.nlm.nih.gov/pubmed/15640462*) have performed an in depth study with regards to this. This study was performed with eight males and eight females of a healthy body weight fasting every other day for 21 days. Partic-ipants lost about $2.5 \pm 0.5\%$ of their body weight including $4 \pm 1\%$ of fat mass over the course of the 21 days. Neither blood glucose nor ghrelin (an appetite hormone) concentrations changed before vs. after the intervention, but insulin concentrations decreased while fasting suggesting greater insulin sensitivity. Study has also suggested that the metabolic machinery required for generating energy from fat was sufficient at the start of the study.

8 Facts About Intermittent Fasting

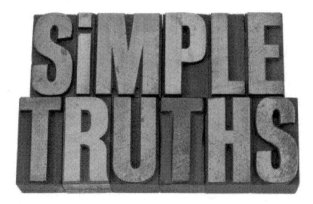

Here are some facts about intermittent fasting that you may not know, but should get familiar with, before you get started.

1. Intermittent Fasting Is Based On Years Of Research

Animal fasting studies date back eighty years. Human fasting studies go back over at least six years. There are increasingly more and more clinical trials being conducted.

2. 'Starvation Mode' Is A Myth

The study that suggested fasting had negative effects was conducted in the 1950's. In this study they took a bunch of young men and asked them to live on approximately half their normal calories and they followed them for six months and they obviously lost dramatic amounts of weight. And when their body fat went down to five percent, they started to experience significant problems. Now that is a really, really radical fast for a really long period of time There was no positive structure to this trial, and the weight loss was done far too quickly. Obviously this then led to negative health issues. Intermittent fasting is nothing like this.

3. Medical Discovery Often Begins With Self-Experimentation

You won't know how a fast can work for *you* until you try it. Everyone is different, everyone is unique, and that is important to keep in mind at all times. What works for others, may not for you. If one fast doesn't suit, try another.

4. Intermittent Fasting Helps You Lose Fat, Not Muscle

A standard diet you lose about 75% fat, 25% muscle. With intermittent fasting, it's between 85 and 100% fat.

5. Not All Fasts Are Created Equal: Intermittent Fasting Is No Juice Fasting

You have to consider *what* you're eating during a fast to ensure that you're including all the food groups. A glass of juice is really just a sugar hit. And that is going to make you feel hungry, it's going to make your insulin levels go up.

6. Dementia Is A Nutrition Issue

The impact of junk food is not just physical. It can have mental affects too. Keep this in mind when selecting the intermittent fast for you, and the foods you eat within that.

7. 'The Fast Diet' Is Still A Work In Progress

There are still studies to be conducted about intermittent fasting. One thing that *has* been determined is that people find it much easier to stick to than other diets. Many test subjects have found it the most successful way to lose fat and keep the weight off.

8. Nothing Has To Hold You Back

You may be worried because of your age, a health condition or something similar, but as long as you speak to a health professional before proceeding – to get some personalized advice – you can be sure that you're doing it in a healthy way.

The Science Behind It

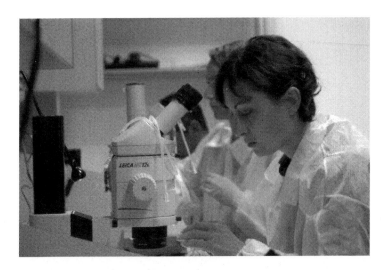

As previously stated, there have been **scientific studies into intermittent fasting**. If this is something that particularly interests you, here is a list to just a few of these:

- Caloric restriction and intermittent fasting: Two potential diets for successful brain aging (*ncbi.nlm.nih.gov/pmc/articles/PMC2622429*). This study demonstrates that fasting can actually help us *slow down the brain aging* process. It concludes that returning to the way that our ancestors used to eat, by fasting, we are actually giving our bodies exactly what they want and need.

- Intermittent fasting dissociates beneficial effects of dietary restriction on glucose metabolism and neuronal resistance to injury from calorie intake (*pnas.org/content/100/10/6216.short*). This study looks at how intermittent fasting affects our hormones, and concludes that it's good for helping us manage illnesses and actually leaves us living a *longer lifespan*.

- Effects of Intermittent Fasting on Serum Lipid Levels, Coagulation Status and Plasma Homocysteine Levels (*karger.com/Article/Abstract/84739*). This study look at what intermittent fasting does to our bodies. It shows that the changes to the serum lipid levels, coagulation status and plasma homocysteine levels is actually really positive and *helps our overall health*.

The next point cover areas in which fasting has **proven benefits**, and the scientific studies that prove this:

1. Brain function

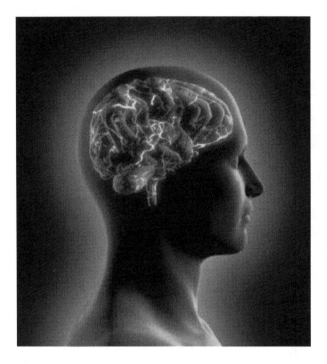

- Fasting boosts neuronal autophagy, which assists it to work properly, at its full potential. The study at *ncbi.nlm.nih.gov/pubmed/20534972* shows the benefits that this therapeutic, neuronal response has on the rest of your body.

- Fasting increases levels of brain-derived neurotrophic factor (BDNF), which is linked to memory and cognitive function. The study at *phys.org/news/2009-02-growth-factor-key-brain-cells.html* shows that fasting helps your brain respond and function faster and more effectively.

- Fasting slows the effects of Huntington's disease. The study (*pnas.org/content/100/5/2911.full*) shows that fasting normalizes blood glucose levels and helps you survive the illness for longer.

- Fasting helps with the brains serotonin content – keeping you happier! The study (*sciencemag.org/content/178/4059/414.short*) shows that fasting allows your brain to produce more serotonin – the hormone that keeps your mood positive.

2. Aging

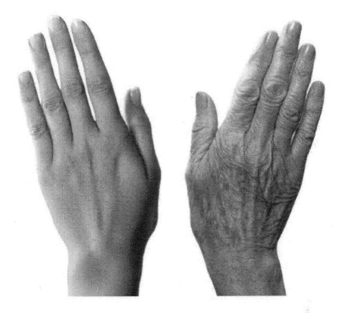

- Fasting is great for helping ward off Alzheimer's. This study (*ncbi.nlm.nih.gov/pubmed/17306982*) shows that fasting helps your brain produce the right chemicals for fighting off Alzheimer's disease.

- Fasting helps your brain age better. The study being referenced (*sciencedirect.com/science/article/pii/S1568163706000523*) shows just how fasting helps your brain remain young. By keeping it working faster and at a higher level, your brain will work more effectively for longer.

- There's evidence that intermittent fasting is good for basic age-related cognitive decline. This study (*ncbi.nlm.nih.gov/pubmed/21861096*) also shows how fasting keeps your cognitive motor function running more successfully and for longer.

3. Disease Prevention

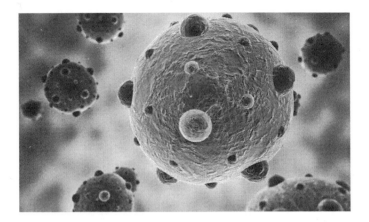

- Fasting increases the production of keytones, which helps protect our bodies against disease. This study (*ncbi.nlm.nih.gov/pubmed/20532550*) shows just how well this keeps our immune systems running.

- Fasting helps prevent the possibility of a stroke. This study (*ncbi.nlm.nih.gov/pmc/articles/PMC2844782*) shows that our brains working more effectively and for longer can help ward off strokes.

- Research indicates that fasting is also effective against physical trauma to the brain. This study (*ncbi.nlm.nih.gov/pubmed/18241053*) demonstrates how fasting can help our brains recover quicker.

- Fasting can help people who suffer from diabetes. This study (*thelancet.com/journals/lancet/article/PIIS0140-6736(10)60484-9/fulltext*) shows that a better control over our diet and when we eat, can actually help diabetes sufferers.

- Fasting can help prevent heart disease. The study being referenced (*thelancet.com/journals/lancet/article/PIIS0140-6736(10)60484-9/fulltext*) helps us see that by controlling when we eat, our bodies and immune systems will look after our hearts better.

- Fasting can help with a cervical spine injury. The study referenced (*ncbi.nlm.nih.gov/pubmed/18585708*) shows that fasting also helps us recover from physical injuries quicker.

4. Wellness

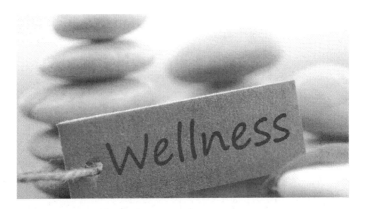

- Fasting helps prevent depression. This study (*scicurious.scientopia.org/2010/12/13/bdnf-and-depression/*) shows that the extra serotonin produced by our brains when fasting, can help us recover from depression.

- Fasting helps regulate your blood glucose levels. This study (*sciencemag.org/content/303/5661/1195.short*) demonstrates how choosing when we eat more carefully, our bodies can produce the glucose levels we need.

- Fasting suppresses the symptoms of a sympathetic nervous system. This study (*sciencemag.org/content/196/4297/1473.short*) shows that fasting increases our norepinephrine hormone when fasting, helping us to ward off issues with our nervous system.

- Fasting actually boosts levels of leptin – making you feel fuller. Whereas some people worry about feeling hungry all the time when fasting, this study (*press.endocrine.org/doi/abs/10.1210/jc.2003-030519*) shows clearly how our bodies work to actually make us feel fuller and more satiated.

Pros And Cons

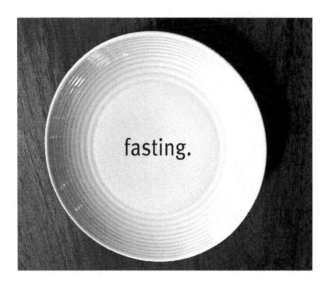

So why should you try intermittent fasting? This chapter looks at the pros and cons of this food plan, to help you make your decision:

Pros

- You'll lose fat, while maintaining muscle.

- Detoxifying your body rids your body of toxins.

- While your body doesn't have to take care of your digestive system, you'll actually end up with more energy.

- Your immune system will also work much more effectively.

Cons

- Your body may need more carbohydrates to run efficiently.

- Your empty stomach can cause issues, such as acid buildup.

If you have any concerns at all, it is always recommended that you speak to a health professional before undertaking a fast. That way you can get advice that's personalized to you and your situation.

Case Studies

The **Daily Fasting Blog** (*www.thedailyfastingblog.com*) is filled with intermittent fasting success stories for you to pour over. Here is an example of one of these:

"Maybe you'll recognize yourself in these paragraphs. Before I began practicing daily intermittent fasting, my day consisted of constant eating. I would often delight in a morning cup of coffee, hot chocolate or tea with cream and sugar. Before lunch time, I would likely have some kind of snack – sometimes a nutritious one like grapes or an apple, and sometimes a not-so-nutritious snack like potato chips, a donut or cookies.

By lunch time, I was ready to eat again and would likely grab a meal from the nearby cafeteria – a sandwich, maybe a salad, and on Fridays, probably an order of fried fish. In the afternoon it was time for another snack to hold me over until I got home. During dinner time I would almost always have seconds, sometimes thirds, and late at night (I'm a night owl) I would snack again on sweets like homemade cookies or bread and/or something savory like nuts, cheese or chips.

Although I enjoyed vegetables like zucchini, broccoli and cabbage, my favorite foods were white rice, bread and beans. I never got tired of those and could, and often did, eat them daily. I didn't indulge in fast food that often, but even when I cooked at home, there was little concern for whether my protein of choice was fried, baked or stewed nor the amount of fat, carbs and calories I was consuming.

In short, I ate whenever and whatever I wanted to eat.

This eating pattern repeated itself over and over again, day after day and along with a mostly sedentary lifestyle working in an office, eventually resulted in my weighing 237 lbs by June 30th, 2014. I knew it wasn't healthy to eat the way I did, but I felt unable to control my appetite even after trying just about every natural appetite suppressant I'd heard of – Sensa, garcinia cambogia, raspberry ketones, and others.

I had tried dieting many times in my life and lost 20, 30, and even 40 pounds on occasion only to gain it all back, and then some. But now I was almost afraid to lose weight for fear of the initial weight-loss only leading to being even heavier in the end. I wasn't fully aware of what I was doing to my body during the surges of calories I was feeding it; and, after a while, I didn't care much. After all, I didn't have diabetes, hypertension, or any major disease and I wasn't on any medication. What was there to be concerned about?

I hadn't always had such a nonchalant attitude about my weight. In 2004 I had lost 40 pounds on the Atkins diet and kept it off for two years only to gradually gain it all back within a year of being off the low-carb wagon. I began to think I should just accept being fat.

Obesity isn't just a cosmetic concern. It increases your risk of diseases and health problems such as heart disease, diabetes and high blood pressure. -The Mayo Clinic website

Later that year, a visit to my doctor for a complete physical confirmed my relatively good health; but, he urged me to lose weight. He told me that at this time in my life – my forties – I was at a critical stage during which obesity greatly increased the odds of acquiring a major health condition within the next several years.

In that moment I thought back to my parents. My dad was diagnosed with diabetes in his mid-forties. My mom was diagnosed with hypertension in her 40's. There was no denying the significant probability of my going down the same path if my lifestyle didn't change.

Still, I didn't know how to do it. I'd tried low-carb dieting as well as low-fat diets with moderate exercise; but despite losing some weight with both, I could never seem to stick to either regimen in the long term. Then, shortly after that physical, a seemingly unrelated activity led to a complete lifestyle change for me.

Although I am not a Muslim, I had always been curious about fasting for Ramadan and admired the commitment and discipline needed to go without food or drink from sunrise to sunset for 30 days. I expressed my curiosity to a few of my Muslim co-workers and they encouraged me to try it. My reasons for exploring Ramadan fasting were not religious, but rather psychological and spiritual. Did I have the self-discipline to subject myself to a period of mindfulness and self-reflection, setting aside a routine of comfort and ease to foster a greater sense of gratitude? That's the question I asked myself as I thought about committing to the 30-day fast.

As the time drew near to start, I was ready to quit my experiment before it began. I recall being scared, nervous and anxious to go without food; but that alone told me that I needed to do it. My co-workers didn't pressure me at all, but I felt a responsibility to at least try it. Still, by the time the start of Ramadan came, I hadn't fasted and didn't intend to do so. That is, until I happened to watch an episode of Naked and Afraid.

As I watched the contestants spend weeks foraging for clean water and food sources much like our ancient ancestors had to do, I suddenly felt no better than a spoiled child unwilling to give up her lollipop. Certainly I could survive less than a day without food or water. After all, if I changed my mind, nourishment was always within arm's reach.

With so much fear and anxiety before starting the fast, I hadn't expected to last a day, but to my surprise, not only did I last to the end of Ramadan, but the longer I fasted, the easier it became. What's more I had indeed learned a lot about myself, and developed a tremendous appreciation for access to clean water and nutritious foods – something I will never take for granted again.

After feeling so good, both physically and mentally, from the effects of fasting for Ramadan, I began exploring the health benefits of fasting and discovered intermittent fasting (IF). I had not fasted for Ramadan to lose weight. As a matter of fact, I had expected to gain weight from feasting at the end of the day. Like many people, I believed one should eat several small meals a day and never skip meals and that doing so was counterproductive to weight-loss. But, I had lost 8 pounds by the end of that month and felt exceptionally energized and in control of my hunger. There were clearly benefits to fasting and as I researched more I learned that there were even more pros than I had first imagined – one of them being weight loss.

I began fasting on June 30, 2014. At that time, I weighed 237 lbs. That's a lot of weight on any woman, but on my 5'5" frame it was dangerous.

As of the writing of this post (a little over three months later), I am 22 lbs. lighter and still working towards my goal of being at a healthy body mass index (BMI). Specifically, my goal is to lose 102 lbs. 92 lbs. by July 1, 2015 and reach my goal weight of 135 lbs. 145 lbs., putting me within a healthy BMI of 24.

So far, daily intermittent fasting, a low-carb (non-ketogenic) diet a healthy diet focused on nutritious home cooked food, and 30 minutes of walking daily has enabled me to lose weight at a moderate steady pace."

Is It Right For You?

From everything you have seen, it's clear why intermittent fasting is so popular. It's a **quick, effective way** to change your life and start to see results. Once you become accustomed to eating according to a planned time, it'll soon feel like an extremely easy lifestyle change.

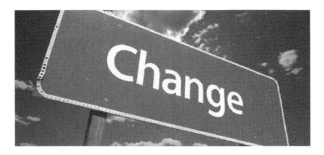

But how do you know **if it's right for you?** You will need to ask yourself a few questions to check that you are in the right place before you begin:

1. What is your **motivation** for doing the fast? Is it strong enough to keep you focused and keep you going?

2. What do you want to **achieve** with the fast?

3. Do you have any **health conditions** that might interfere? Should you consult your doctor first?

4. Are there any **obstacles** that are likely to crop up and throw you off course during the first few weeks? If so, this may prevent you from forming the fasting habit that will carry you through.

If you feel that you are ready, and that you're prepared to put in the necessary dedication, then now is the time to start. If you go into it with a haphazard attitude, you're setting yourself up for failure.

So **which type of fasting do you choose?** Well, the next chapter will cover the top 10 fasting protocols for you to get an idea of which diet is best for you, but you really need to think about what your end goal is – is it weight loss, muscle building, a healthier lifestyle, or something else. You'll also need to really consider what is possible. There is no point in you choosing a fast that is going to clash with your job or your lifestyle, or it's going to quickly become unmanageable. So read on to find a fast that's right for you.

TOP 10 INTERMITTENT FASTING PROTOCOLS

Now that you know a little bit more about intermittent fasting – including examples – it's time to delve into protocols, to help you decide which intermittent fast is best for you. The next chapter of this book will give you some sample diets for each protocol, so once you've decided; you can get started with the protocol of your choice.

1. Three Day Fast

This fast can be done as often as required. A lot of people, who are just starting out with fasting, decide to begin with this to see how they get on. However, you consume zero calories during this time – drinking only water, so if 3 days seems a little overwhelming, you *can* reduce this to 24 or 48 hours.

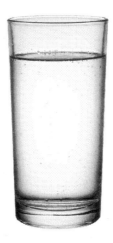

Recommended For: Beginners – those wanting to see how their body will cope with a fast.

How It Works: You will *only* drink water during this time. No solid foods or other liquids are to be consumed. Aim to drink between 1 and a half and 3 liters of water in one day – zero calories in total. You will need to pick a time to do this when you're able to cope with any side effects. An overly busy period filled with stress and deadlines would be the worst time to attempt this diet – especially for the very first time.

Pros: You will cleanse your system and give your digestive system a much needed rest. You will also notice weight loss during this time period.

Cons: You my experience some unpleasant side effects – dizziness, nausea, etc. You may also experience bouts of hunger, but you can counteract this by drinking a couple of glasses of water.

This can be a great way to get yourself started by trying fasting with less pressure, in a shorter burst – that way you'll begin to learn how your body reacts before making any further decisions. It's always advisable to get advice from a health professional before starting any fast, particularly if it's your first one, so you can get some personalized advice that suits your situation.

2. LeanGains

We've already had a little look at LeanGains, but here is a little more information about the process involved.

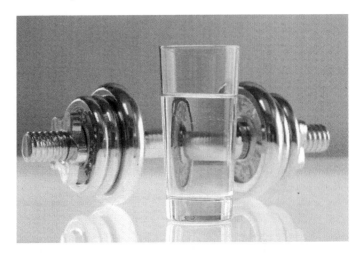

Recommended For: Dedicated gym-goers, who want to lose body fat and build muscle.

How It Works: Women fast for 14 hours, men for 16. During the fasting period, only black coffee, calorie-free sweeteners, diet soda, water and sugar-free gum are permitted. You'll not want to consume any calories. This is more easily achieved when you include the hours in which you're sleeping. The remaining 8 to 10 hours are the time where you're eating, and during this period you'll want to select your foods carefully, to ensure that you're eating the right things to allow you to continue exercising.

What and when you eat depends entirely on your workout schedule. On the days you exercise, including carbohydrates in your meals is more important than fat. If you have rest days, make sure your fat intake is higher, and protein needs to be high every day.

To work out exactly **how many calories** you should be eating **during the non-fasting time** on the LeanGains diet, it's recommended that you use the ***Harris-Benedict equation***. The formula for this is as follows:

Men: BMR = 88.362 + (13.397 x weight kg) + (4.799 x height cm) - (5.677 x age years)

Women: BMR = 447.593 + (9.247 x weight kg) + (3.098 x height cm) -

(4.330 x age years)

Let's look at an example of this, to help you with working out your own. For this example, let's say that you're a 30-year-old male, with a weight of 76kg and a height of 180cm. This would look like this:

88. 362 + (13.397 x 76) + (4.799 x 180) - (5.677 x 30) = 1800

So this would give you a BMR (Basal Metabolic Rate) of 1800. This amount tells the amount of calories you would burn if you were asleep all day. This way you can work out the number of daily calories you need per day to maintain the weight you're at by simply multiplying the BRM with PAL (Your Physical Activity Level).

If this is something that's too complex to work out on your own, there are a number of online tools that can assist you in working out your number, such as **Many Tools** at *manytools.org/handy/bmr-calculator/*. Using the example above, not only does it show the BMR of 1800, it gives a daily calorie amount of 2700.

Measuring sytem:	Metric (cm/Kg) ▾
Height (centimeters):	180
Weight (Kg):	76
Age:	30
Gender:	Male ▾
Activity level:	Moderately physical work, no exercise (1.5) ▾

Calculate!

Your BMR

BMR: **1800**
Daily Calorie Needs: **2700 calories**.

Calculation based on the revised Harris-Benedict equation by Roza and Shizgal from 1984.
PAL (Physical activity level): 1.5
Gender: male

If weight loss is your end goal, you can then reduce this amount as follows – the guideline is simply there to help you exercise and diet at the same time.

Pros: A lot of people feel that the flexibility of *when* you eat is of benefit. You can choose to split your meals up into three, or eat as you wish during your eight-hour "feeding" period.

Cons: LeanGains *does* have a lot of guidelines on *what* to eat, to fit in with your workout. Some people find this challenging to work with as they'd prefer the flexibility about what to consume that comes with other fasting protocols. You can learn more about the specifics - as well as when to time these meals - directly from Leangains at *www.leangains.com*.

People who are dedicated to working out, generally think a lot about what they eat anyway. They often know exactly how much of each food category that they need to maintain the body that they need. They also often know a lot about the supplements that help their diet along (and area that we look at in the following chapter). When they undertake this protocol, all they really need to think about is moving about the times that they eat these foods. However, if this is something that you'd like to look into further, check out **Ripped Body** (*rippedbody.jp*). This website is filled with useful tips about the best things to eat while fasting, to ensure the end result is increased muscle mass.

3. Eat Stop Eat

This has also been discussed a little, earlier on in the book. But more details are included here.

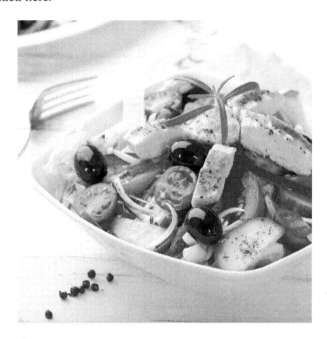

Recommended For: Healthy eaters looking for an extra boost.

How It Works: This fast is all about moderation. You can still eat what you want, but maybe not as much of it. The fasting periods are for 24 hours, twice a week. No calories are consumed during this time, but afterwards you can resume eating as normal.

Here is an example of the amount of calories that Brad Pilon – the creator of the diet – suggests that you should eat on a weekly basis, splitting the fast into 2 parts (which some may find a better way to do it):

- Monday – Eat 900 calories then start fasting

- Tuesday – End fasting then eat 1400 calories

- Wednesday – Eat 1800 calories

- Thursday – Eat 1800 calories

- Friday – Eat 900 calories then start fasting

- Saturday – End fasting and eat 1200 calories

- Sunday – Eat 1800 calories

As this amount is much less than what you'd normally consume, it's best to really think about what you are eating, to get the most out of your calories. Sure, you could eat a bar of chocolate – but that will take up a large chunk of your daily limit. It'll be good to familiarize yourself with a calorie calculating tool, such as Calorie Counter, until you get used to counting your daily amount for yourself.

Pros: While 24 hours may seem like a long time to go without food, the good news is that this program is flexible. You don't have to go all-or-nothing at the beginning. Go as long as you can without food the first day and gradually increase fasting phase over time to help your body adjust.

Cons: This is very likely to be a struggle at the beginning. You may experience symptoms such as headaches, fatigue, or feeling cranky or anxiety. You will also need a degree of self-control to ensure you don't binge immediately after the fast.

This diet will *really* get you thinking about exactly what you're putting into your body, making it extremely good for your health. When you start paying attention to consuming a more balanced diet, you will start to reap the benefits. Here are some examples of **what you can get from eating a balanced diet:**

- **Controls your weight** – maintaining a healthy weight brings with it a lot of other benefits. You will look and feel much better.

- **Your mood will improve** – not only will you have a higher self-esteem, feeling better in yourself will also have positive mental effects.

- **Combats diseases** – eating right helps manage your blood pressure, your cholesterol and your blood flow. To name just a few, you'll reduce your risk of heart disease, a stroke and certain types of cancer.

- **Boosts your energy levels** – experiencing less of that lethargic feeling will leave you free to get much more done in a day. You will also sleep better, leaving you feeling much more refreshed.

- **Improves longevity** – eating right will give you a much better chance of living longer.

4. The Warrior Diet

The Warrior Diet is a higher level of fasting – for the more experienced faster. Only try this if you know exactly how your body is going to react to long periods of not eating.

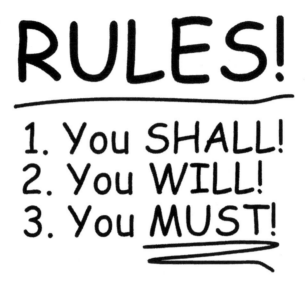

RULES!

1. You SHALL!
2. You WILL!
3. You MUST!

Recommend For: People who like following rules. This is for those who find structure much easier to cope with.

How It Works: With this diet, you will fast for 20 hours a day, eating one big meal at night. What you eat within this meal is key to its success. During the fasting period, you *can* eat raw vegetables and fruit, fresh juice and a few servings of protein if desired. It's more about under-eating, rather than not eating at all.

To work out how many calories you need to eat on this diet, use the *Harris-Benedict equation* discussed previously in this chapter. The only difference with this diet is that you'll want to consume the majority of these calories in one meal.

It's also important to think about what you're going to eat with this meal. Where you'll be eating raw products throughout the day, you will want to be sure to include protein, carbohydrates and dairy with your meal. There are also Warrior products available on the market, to make your diet much easier. Defense Nutrition (*www.defensenutrition.com*) has a great selection available.

Pros: Being able to snack during the fasting period can make it easier to get through.

Cons: There are strict guidelines to what you eat, which can make it difficult to maintain – especially when it comes to socializing.

It's likely that you'll need to give this diet a try before settling on it. Consuming just one main meal per day is a big commitment. However, the pay off of doing this successfully can be huge:

- It boosts your metabolism.

- You see an improvement in overall health – from vitality to virility.

- Your lean muscle mass increases.

- It's proven to slow the aging process.

5. Fat Loss Forever

This plan takes the best parts of the 3 plans listed above. It's been designed to mix up the hours of fasting to suit individualized needs – which means it's great because it can fit around you. It boasts that it's perfect for people who work long shifts because it's so adaptable to anyone's needs.

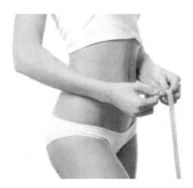

Recommended For: People who need flexibility in their fasting protocols.

How It Works: With this plan, you will fast for varying amounts of hours each day. You'll even get one cheat day, which is followed by a 36 hour fast. The full details of how to divvy up the rest of the fasting hours can be found at the website of the creator of this diet – **Omega Blue Print** at *bit.ly/omega_body_blueprint*. For this diet, you will need to sign up to the website to get your personalized nutrition and exercise recommendations. You *will* need to be dedicated and have a clear end goal for this plan, because the advice from the trainers does not come free. However, the calorie amounts set will give you results because the plan has been made just for you.

Pros: The varying fasting hours can fit around your chaotic, busy lifestyle. This diet has been designed to fit around *you*, proving that everyone can do an intermittent fast.

Cons: You will have to pay for this plan, because it's so tailored to you. Here is a sample of one of the '500 calorie' days, to give you an idea of what your plan might look like:

- Vegetables – 1 serving, 2 times a day
- Fruits – 1 serving, 2 times a day
- 100gm lean meat, 2 times a day

- 2 Thin Sunrice Rice Cakes or 2 melba toasts or 2 grissini breadsticks – daily

- The juice of one lemon each day (optional)

- Fresh herbs and spices– unlimited

If intermittent fasting is something that you are *really* committed to, then this is a diet that's definitely worth considering. The Internet is filled with rave reviews about this diet from real people that have tried it, such as this from Critical Bench (*criticalbench.com/fatloss-forever-review*):

"I'm happy to say that John and Dan have put together an excellent program that presents a solid foundation for effective fat loss. The guys use a straightforward approach that's easy to follow and not difficult to read. For anyone who has been frustrated in his efforts to shed unwanted fat, you ought to consider the FLF approach—it's built on solid science that can deliver the desired results!"

6. UpDayDownDay Diet

The theory behind this diet is simple. Eat very little one day, then like normal the next. It's also sometimes referred to as *alternate day fasting*.

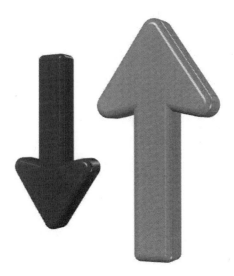

Recommended For: Disciplined dieters with a specific goal weight. This will be a challenge at first, but in a study conducted by Dr. Varaday, it was found that people found it easier to follow the diet after approximately 10 days.

"It takes about a week to 10 days or so to get used to that up-down pattern of eating. But it's amazing. Even though people struggle through the first week, they always say, 'After a week, I had no problem eating just 500 calories every other day."

How It Works: As stated previously, this diet is all about eating normally one day, and consuming a reduced amount of calories the next. On the low calorie days, you will eat a fifth of your normal intake. So 2,000 calories will become 400, and 2,500 calories will become 500. Meal replacement shakes can help you with the low calorie days, and keep workouts to the 'normal' days to ensure that you get the most out of your exercise.

When following this diet, it's important to organize your calories well – on the fasting and non-fasting days. It's suggested that you always think about:

- *Healthy fats.* Try to get at least 50% of your daily calories from healthy fats, such as avocados, organic grass-fed butter, pastured egg yolks, coconut oil, and raw nuts such as macadamia, pecans, and pine nuts.

- *Protein* – 40 to 80 grams per day will be plenty to keep you healthy. Try to ensure that you're getting your meat from organically raised, grass-fed or pastured animals.

- *Fresh, raw vegetables* – you can eat as many of these as you like per day.

Pros: This method is great for weight loss. It also promotes a much healthier lifestyle as you'll need to get the most out of your calorie limit.

Cons: It can be challenging not to binge on 'normal' days. Plan ahead to help yourself with this – setting yourself a food schedule will help you stick to it.

When thinking about your non fasting days on this diet, you don't want to go over the top and completely negate all the good work that you've done on you fasting days. You will be more successful with reaching your goals, if you set yourself a strict calorie level for all days, and stick to it.

7. Food For Thought

This is sometimes known as the *5:2 Fast*, where five days of the week are spent eating normally, and two are reduced calorie, fasting days.

Recommended For: Those who need some flexibility within their fasting days. You can choose your own two days per week to fast, so you can fit it around anything that crops up.

How It Works: For 5 days a week, women can consume up to 2,000 calories per day and men 2,400. On the 2 fasting days, women can eat 500 and men 600, although you *can* get a more specified recommendation of this from a health professional, depending on your BMI and activity level.

Here are some **tips for the sort of things you should be eating** on this diet:

- Carbohydrates aren't good for fasting days. They will use up most of your calories.

- Fruits, vegetables, salads and small servings of protein are good calories.

- Added herbs, spices and flavorings are good for making things taste more exciting.

- Soups are also a good filler food.

- Many people who have tried the 5:2 diet have found that on fasting days, it's better to skip breakfast and eat later on. Although it's advisable to experiment with eating times to see what suits you best. You can even go from 3 meals to 2.

- Fresh, raw ingredients are the best to eat on this diet. Select the in-season ones for the tastiest food.

- Have something instant to hand in case of a snack attack: if you love sweet things, then no-sugar jelly is ideal at less than 10 calories.

- Drink lots – fill yourself on water, tea and coffee (remembering to count the calories in milk).

- Here are some useful food swapping tips to help you along the way too:

  o Swap bananas for fresh or frozen berries in yogurt, for less of a sugar rebound.

  o Swap quiches or flans for omelets – all the flavor, none of the high-calorie pastry.

  o Swap high-fat hard cheeses for lower-fat ricotta, feta or reduced fat cream cheese.

  o Swap cappuccino for a black Americano.

  o Swap ice cream for home-made lollies (made from low-sugar cordials and berries).

  o Swap rice for cauliflower 'rice' – grate a portion of uncooked cauliflower and microwave for 1-2 minutes for a lower-calorie substitute.

  o Swap tagliatelle for courgettes sliced into thin ribbons with a potato peeler – boil or steam for 1 minute and serve with your normal pasta sauce.

Pros: It can quickly become a lifestyle change for you, because you can select the 2 fasting days according to your weekly plan – eating as normal on the other days, so business, socializing and working out won't get in the way.

Cons: It can be challenging not to overeat on the 5 'normal' days. You will want to ensure that you don't waste calories on eating quick fix junk food that won't leave you feeling full.

This is another diet that really gets you thinking about what you're eating to ensure that you're not wasting calories. On the fasting days, your body will go into 'repair mode' and any damaged cells inside of your body will repair themselves. This intermittent fast will allow you reap all of the health benefits of intermittent fasting, in an extremely manageable way.

8. Spontaneous Meal Skipping

This is also referred to as mini fasting, and is a much more relaxed attitude to fasting. It's all about working out *exactly* when you're hungry, and avoiding meals when you aren't. This plan isn't set in stone or scheduled, so you can fit it around any plans. Becoming more in tune with your body will allow you to see just how much you over eat.

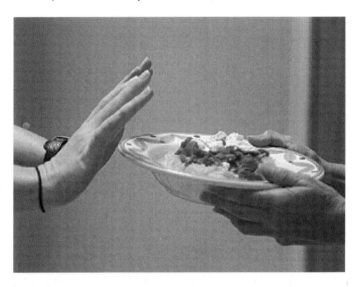

Recommended For: People with extremely busy and chaotic lifestyle, who want to fast but cannot find a way to fit it in.

How It Works: As long as you are sure to eat healthy, then it's possible to perform intermittent fasting by skipping meals when you're busy, not hungry or able to have a food break. In fact, Mercola suggests that two meals per day can actually be much better than more.

"Longo says studies that support a grazing approach tend to be flawed in predictable ways. They often look only at the short-term effects of increasing meal frequency.

While your appetite, metabolism, and blood sugar might at first improve, your system will grow accustomed to your new eating schedule after a month or two. When that happens, your body will start expecting and craving food all day long instead of only around midday or dinnertime."

The **health benefits** that you can receive from giving this a try are as follows:

- It'll limit inflammation; reduce oxidative stress, and cellular damage.

- It'll improve circulating glucose.

- It'll improve metabolic efficiency and body composition, including significant reductions in body weight in obese individuals.

- It'll reduce LDL and total cholesterol levels.

- It will help prevent or reverse type 2 diabetes, as well as slow its progression.

- It will improve immune function and shift stem cells from a dormant state to a state of self-renewal.

- It'll improve pancreatic function.

- It'll improve insulin and leptin levels and insulin/leptin sensitivity.

- You'll notice a reduced blood pressure.

- It will reproduce some of the cardiovascular benefits associated with physical exercise.

- It'll help protect against cardiovascular disease.

- It'll modulate levels of dangerous visceral fat.

- It will boost mitochondrial energy efficiency.

- It'll help normalize ghrelin levels, known as "the hunger hormone".

- It will help eliminate sugar cravings as your body adapts to burning fat instead of sugar.

- It will help promote human growth hormone production (HGH).

- It will boost production of brain-derived neurotrophic factor (BDNF), stimulating the release of new brain cells and triggering brain chemicals that protect against changes associated with Alzheimer's and Parkinson's disease.

So as you can see, there are a number of health benefits you can receive from eating when you're hungry rather than grazing constantly. You may also want to look into ensuring that you get a **balanced diet** when you *are* eating to keep yourself healthy. Here are some great tips on this:

- Eat at least five portions of fruit and vegetables a day. If you can, try to include more.

- Cut down your sugar and saturated fat intake.

- Drink plenty of water, six to eight glasses are the recommended amount.

- Aim for at least two portions of fish every week.

- Reduce your salt intake. It is advised to eat no more than 6g a day. Avoid adding it to your meals, you'll be surprised at how much is already there.

- Use starchy foods as the base of your meals. These act as your fuel for the day.

Pros: There is no pressure with this diet. It all depends on what you feel it best to do. The great thing about this diet is that you will get used to exactly what you want and need at all times. Knowing your body better, can only be a good thing.

Cons: It can take longer to see results, and the relaxed attitude can make it harder to stick to, however if you're dedicated enough you can make a real difference.

Some people find this a lot easier to stick to, others struggle. The most important thing is making it work for you. Again, this is *much* easier if you're eating healthier, as junk food isn't filled with any of the right nutrition that leaves us sated. Consuming it leads us to a crash, which results in us eating more!

9. Natural Nightly Fasting

There is another easy fasting method which is perfect for beginners. This plan is all about **fasting at night** – when we sleep – and in the evenings. This is an extremely natural method, which can fit into almost any lifestyle.

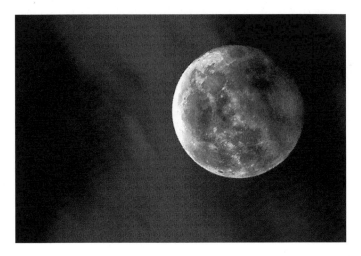

Recommended For: Beginners – this is a natural way to introduce yourself to fasting. A lot of diets recommend avoiding food at night, this is simply a more structured way of doing this.

How It Works: This is a way of fasting by avoiding eating in the evenings. The only thing you really need to do is ensure that there is a 10 to 12-hour period where you consume nothing – including the time that you're asleep. The amount of calories that you should eat during the non-fasting time can be found using the *Harris-Benedict equation*, discussed previously.

The great thing about this diet is that you can keep up your exercise regime. If this is the case, here is some advice on the sort of **foods that you should eat before workout out**:

- Low fat
- Moderate in carbohydrates and protein
- Low fiber
- Includes fluids
- Made up of familiar foods that you tolerate well

Pros: This is easy to turn into an effective lifestyle change that will show results. Because it's not a strict diet, you will find the results much easier to maintain.

Cons: It may take longer to see these results, but it'll be worth it in the long run. You will also need to be careful about what you're eating during the day. The better you eat, the easier you will find this to keep up.

This diet plan comes with all of the benefits of intermittent fasting, without having too much of an impact on your life. You can still consume three meals a day, with the normal amount of calories that you should be eating per day, just nothing in the evening. It's a great way to give fasting a go.

10. Carb Backloading

This is an intermittent fast style that helps you workout. It includes intermittent fasting and the right diet to ensure that you continue to build muscle. This is great for creating a muscular and lean body because maintaining muscle is great for raising your metabolism.

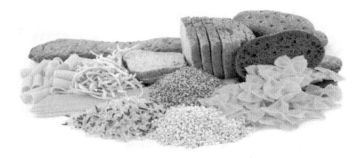

Recommended For: Those who want to build muscle as they fast. This diet proves that fasting is not only for losing weight.

How It Works: You fast for 8 hours a day, using the remaining 16 to eat. During this time, you consume all of your proteins and fats in the morning, saving most of the carbohydrates and calories for the evening after you have worked out.

Here are some tips on getting this diet right:

- Use supplements, such as protein powder and omega 3, to help you with your fast.
- Fast overnight and in the morning for the best results.
- Save the majority of your daily carbohydrates for after your workout for the best results.
- Ensure that you're sleeping pattern is regular for an easier fast.
- Use caffeine for a necessary boost.

Pros: This diet is great for bodybuilders and those that like to work out a lot, because the fast won't affects your program, and helps you to effectively continue to build your muscle.

Cons: This plan *does* take a lot of scheduling as you'll need to work it around your exercise regime. However, with the right plan in place, you will quickly see results.

Now you have seen some of the most commonly used fasting methods, you may now have some idea about which protocol would be the most effective and beneficial for you. This should give you some idea of what plan fits in more with your current lifestyle and end goals.

The next chapter goes on to look more about tips for getting you started with your fast. It will cover the six most important things to think about when getting started.

6 ULTIMATE STEPS FOR GETTING STARTED

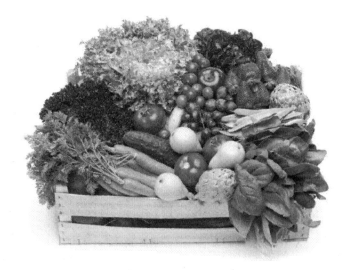

1. Determine your goals and pick a fast accordingly.

As much as it's important to fit the fast in with your lifestyle, it's vital that you also think about what you want to get out of the fast. If you're unhappy with the results, it's unlikely that you'll continue with the lifestyle change that you've begun – wasting all of your efforts.

When looking at your goals, it's always advisable to use the **SMART** acronym:

- **S**pecific

- **M**easurable

- **A**ttainable

- **R**ealistic

- **T**ime-bound.

An example of creating a SMART goal for your fast would work like this:

Such as '*I want to lose weight*'.

- **Specific** – You will need to make this more specific. *'I want to lose 10 pounds'*.

- **Measurable** – How are you going to ensure that you keep up with this? 'I will follow the 5 2 fast – choosing Monday and Thursday as my fast days'.

- **Attainable** – Is this possible? Are Mondays and Thursdays always going to be suitable? Do you have a backup plan if not? *'Wednesday will be my backup day'*.

- **Realistic** – Are you *really* going to be able to stick to the 500/600 calories on the 2 fast days? Will you be able to eat healthily in between? If you're unsure, you should consult your doctor for advice before starting. *'I will test myself with a 24 hour fast first'*.

- **Time-bound** – You will want to keep an eye on your progress, to check that you're heading towards your goal. *'I will weight myself weekly'*.

Setting goals in this way has proven benefits and will help you meet them. They are much more structured, clearly possible and leave nothing to hold you back. Print out this information and store it somewhere clear for you to see every day. Make yourself accountable for your own plan.

Once you have decided on the goal you wish to aim for, it's time to choose a fast to suit this. We have already looked at some of the most common fasting protocols in the previous chapter, but if this is something that you'd like to look at in more detail, here are some resources for you:

The IF Life at *theiflife.com*

Precision Nutrition at *precisionnutrition.com/intermittent-fasting/summary*

Ultimate Paleo Guide at *ultimatepaleoguide.com/intermittent-fasting-protocols*

Muscle For Life at *muscleforlife.com/the-definitive-guide-to-intermittent-fasting*

Roman Fitness Systems at *romanfitnesssystems.com/articles/intermittent-fasting-201*

2. Select the best time to begin and the most effective number of meals to suit this.

Once you have worked out which plan you want to follow, you'll need to work out the most suitable hours to abstain from food to suit yourself. You'll likely want to include the hours you're sleeping in the fast – so that makes it a *little* easier. The rest of it will have to be worked out around your lifestyle and work.

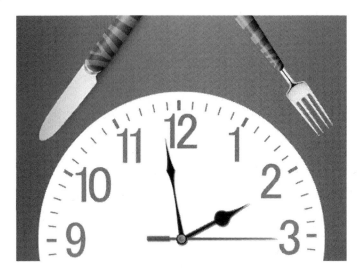

Some fasts have a dictation on how many meals or snacks you should eat per day. Others are more varied and leave the choice up to you. So should you have one or two meals, or 5 or 6 snacks? Because of the limited time, and because it's the way we usually work, most people select to have up to 3 meals per day. This is also a more effective method as it gives your body a chance to digest food more effectively.

3. Decide on foods to include.

One of the most common questions asked about fasting is *'what can I eat?'* A lot of the diets don't specify, but it can be difficult to know what *'eat as normal'* means on your non-fasting days. It can also be a challenge to get the most out of your allowed calories on your fasting days. You still want to get everything that you need to be able to function properly.

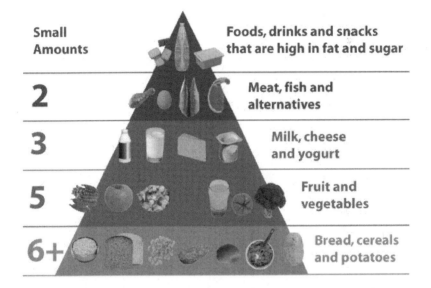

Small Amounts	**Foods, drinks and snacks that are high in fat and sugar**
2	**Meat, fish and alternatives**
3	**Milk, cheese and yogurt**
5	**Fruit and vegetables**
6+	**Bread, cereals and potatoes**

Now we will look at all of the diets for the protocols we've talked about in the previous chapter, with samples of what you can actually eat while doing them.

24 HOUR FAST

The first diet shown was the three-day fast, but you can also do a 24-hour fast to begin with. Of course, during this time, you eat nothing. However, if you'd like to ease yourself in with a sample, then follow these guidelines:

Calories: 0 – 300 (max) fasting day, 2,000 on non-fasting days.

Macronutrients: Protein is the most important element on the fasting day, but all the macronutrients (proteins, fats and carbohydrates) are consumed in moderation on the rest of the days.

- 10 PM the day before fast:
  o Eat your last meal of the day.
  o Drink 500ml (2 cups) of water.
- 10 AM fasting day:
  o Drink 1L (4 cups) of water + 1 serving greens powder
  o Drink 250ml (1 cup) of green tea.
  o Take 5 grams Branched Chain Amino Acids Powder.
- 3 PM:
  o Drink 1L (4 cups) of water + 1 serving greens powder.
  o Drink 250ml (1 cup) green tea.
  o Take 5 grams Branched Chain Amino Acids powder.
- 10 PM:
  o Eat a small snack before bed.
  o Drink 500ml (2 cups) of water.

For your small snack, include something that is high in protein, but less than 300 calories, e.g. a tablespoon of almond butter and some celery. For this diet, the least amount of calories consumed in the 24-hour period, the better. Remember that drinking water in particular helps to mitigate feelings of hunger. After this, you will return to non-fasting days, in which you'll consume the recommended amount of calories set by the *Harris-Benedict equation.*

You will also notice that **supplements** have been mentioned here. These are often used to ensure that we're getting everything we need during a fast.

They are not essential to fasting, but they make it a lot of easier. On top of the ones mentioned above, below are some supplements that might just make your fasting journey easier – whatever diet plan you're following:

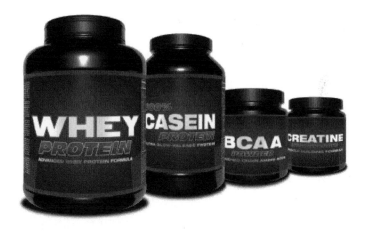

- Multivitamin – an easy way to safeguard against any deficiencies.
- Fish Oil – helps keep your Omega 3 and 6 levels up.
- Calcium – increases fat excretion and boosts testosterone.
- Vitamin D – helps you function optimally.
- Branched Chain Amino Acids (BCAA) - can help limit lean body mass loss as well as increasing visceral fat loss.
- Creatine – helps boost muscle (when working out).
- Beta Alanine – boosts exercise performance.
- Whey Protein – protein boost for pre and post workout.
- Casein Protein – ideal for pre bedtime.
- Glucosamine – ideal for relieving joint pain.
- Caffeine – if you don't drink coffee, this can give you a necessary energy boost to keep you going.

But **what should you eat on the non-fasting days?** You want to ensure that you're getting everything that you need. Here is an example menu to give you some ideas about what you could eat. You could use some of these meals for the remaining 6 week days after your 24 hour fast:

DAY 1:

Breakfast: 1 toasted whole wheat English muffin with 1 Tbsp. fruit spread, 1 hard-boiled egg and 1 orange.

- calories - 390
- fat - 6 grams
- saturated fat - 1.5 grams
- carbohydrates - 54 grams
- cholesterol - 185 mg
- fiber - 8 grams
- sodium - 290 mg

Lunch: Bean burrito.

- calories - 221
- fat - 3 grams
- saturated fat - 1.5 grams
- carbohydrates - 45 grams
- cholesterol - 7 mg
- fiber - 9 grams
- sodium - 800 mg

Dinner: 3 ounces baked white fish with lemon juice, 1 cup zucchini and 1 cup red peppers and 1 small baked potato.

- calories - 400
- fat - 8 grams
- saturated fat - 1 gram
- carbohydrates - 52 grams
- cholesterol - 63 mg
- fiber - 8 grams
- sodium - 225 mg

DAY 2:

Breakfast: 3/4 cup cooked plain oatmeal, prepared with 1/2 cup skim milk, with 1/2 cup chopped apple and 2 tablespoons raisins.

- calories - 270
- fat - 1 gram
- saturated fat - 0 grams
- carbohydrates - 60 grams
- cholesterol - 0 mg
- fiber - 7 grams
- sodium - 75 mg

Lunch: chicken sandwich on whole grain bread, with light mayonnaise, lettuce, and tomato, 1 cup non-fat fruited yogurt and 1/2 cup canned peaches or granola.

- calories - 450
- fat - 8 grams
- saturated fat - 1.5 grams
- carbohydrates - 68 grams
- cholesterol - 60 mg
- fiber - 11 grams
- sodium - 450 mg

Dinner: Vegetarian chili

- calories - 130
- fat - 1 gram
- saturated fat - 0 grams
- carbohydrates - 23 grams
- cholesterol - 10 mg
- fiber - 8 grams

- sodium - 160 mg

DAY 3:

Breakfast: 2 eggs scrambled (or 1/2 cup egg substitute), 1 slice whole wheat toast with 1 teaspoon trans-fat free margarine and 1 small fresh pear (or seasonal fruit)

- calories - 340
- fat - 14 gram
- saturated fat - 3.5 grams
- carbohydrates - 40 grams
- cholesterol - 370 mg
- fiber - 7 grams
- sodium - 430 mg

Lunch: 1 cup minestrone, side salad with 1 tablespoon low-fat dressing, 1 slice whole grain toast with 1 teaspoon margarine.

- calories - 306
- fat - 8 grams
- saturated fat - 1 gram
- carbohydrates - 35 grams
- cholesterol - 56 mg
- fiber - 12 grams
- sodium - 345 mg

Dinner: 1 1/3 cup beef stroganoff, 1 cup cooked cauliflower and broccoli with 1 tablespoon shredded cheese.

- calories - 550
- fat - 9.5 grams
- saturated fat - 3.5 grams
- carbohydrates - 75 grams

- cholesterol - 55 mg
- fiber - 8 grams
- sodium - 360 mg

DAY 4:

Breakfast: 1 cup whole grain cold cereal with 1/2 cup skim milk and 1/2 banana.

- calories - 206
- fat - 1 gram
- saturated fat - 0 gram
- carbohydrates - 44 grams
- cholesterol - 0 mg
- fiber - 75grams
- sodium - 270 mg

Lunch: Vegetarian chili (leftover from Day 2 dinner).

- calories - 130
- fat - 1 gram
- saturated fat - 0 grams
- carbohydrates - 23 grams
- cholesterol - 10 mg
- fiber - 8 grams
- sodium - 160 mg

Dinner: 3 ounces baked chicken breast, skin removed, 1/2 cup brown or wild rice and 1/2 cup cooked carrots mixed with frozen peas.

- calories - 510
- fat - 21 grams
- saturated fat - 3.5 grams
- carbohydrates - 45 grams

- cholesterol - 72 mg
- fiber - 9 grams
- sodium - 200 mg

DAY 5:

Breakfast: 2 slices of whole wheat French toast topped with two teaspoons of unsweetened applesauce mixed with 1 tablespoon maple syrup and 8 ounces of non-fat fruited yogurt.

- calories - 422
- fat - 10 grams
- saturated fat - 2 grams
- carbohydrates - 65 grams
- cholesterol - 5 mg
- fiber - 4 grams
- sodium - 540 mg

Lunch: 1 cup low-fat cottage cheese topped with 1/2 cup fruit cocktail, baby carrots and cherry tomatoes with 1/4 cup low-fat ranch dressing and 1 slice whole wheat bread with 1 teaspoon 100% fruit spread.

- calories - 500
- fat - 14 grams
- saturated fat - 2.5 grams
- carbohydrates - 55 grams
- cholesterol - 15 mg
- fiber - 5 grams
- sodium - 560 mg

Dinner: 1 cup whole wheat spaghetti with turkey meatballs (meatballs made with ground turkey instead of ground beef) and a side salad.

- calories - 510
- total fat - 21 grams

- saturated fat - 3.5 grams

- carbohydrates - 45 grams

- cholesterol - 72 mg

- fiber - 9 grams

- sodium - 200 mg

DAY 6:

Breakfast: 1 slice whole wheat toast with 1 tablespoon peanut butter, 1 cup non-fat fruited yogurt and 1 fresh orange.

- calories - 360

- fat - 10 grams

- saturated fat - 2 grams

- carbohydrates - 57 grams

- cholesterol - 5 mg

- fiber - 7 grams

- sodium - 340 mg

Lunch: 3 ounces tuna (either canned in water or in fresh pouch) with light mayonnaise, 2-3 pieces of lettuce and tomato on 2 slices of whole wheat or whole grain bread, 1 small apple and 1 cup low-fat, low-sodium cottage cheese.

- calories - 464

- fat - 6 grams

- saturated fat - 1 gram

- carbohydrates - 60 grams

- cholesterol - 57 mg

- fiber - 10 grams

- sodium - 830 mg

Dinner: Veggie fajitas and1 1/2 cups spinach salad and fat-free dressing.

- calories - 408
- fat - 15 grams
- saturated fat - 2 grams
- carbohydrates - 62 grams
- cholesterol - 0 mg
- fiber - 14 grams
- sodium - 405 mg

THREE-DAY FAST

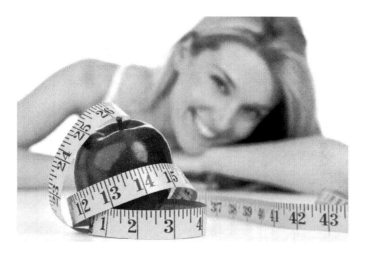

Three-day fast is an extended 24-hour fast, hence you can reuse the same recommendations for your fasting days as from the chapter above.

Consider this diet if it's your first ever fast. This will make things much easier and will still help you lose 10 pounds a week by keeping your metabolism at its current levels.

Calories: 500 – 600 on fasting days (anything less than 1000 calories is considered as fasting), and 1500 on non-fasting days. Alternatively use a 0-300 calorie restriction for fasting days as for 24-hour fasting discussed above.

Macronutrients: This diet ensures that you get all of the protein and fats that you need, minimizing the carbohydrates quantity. It's a combination of low calorie, chemically compatible foods designed to work together and jump start your weight loss.

DAY 1 of Fasting:

- Breakfast
    - o 1/2 Grapefruit – it kick starts the liver into fat burning mode
    - o 1 Slice of whole wheat Toast or 1/8 cup of sunflower seeds or 1/2 cup of whole grain cereal.
    - o 2 Tablespoons of Peanut Butter or Almond butter – high protein foods require more energy from the body to process, so they burn more fat to digest.

- o   1 cup Coffee or Green Tea (with caffeine) – caffeine raises the metabolism slightly, helping your body lose weight by burning fat.

- Lunch
    - o   1/2 Cup of Tuna or 1 cup of cottage cheese
    - o   1 Slice of Toast or 2 rice cakes
    - o   1 cup Coffee or Green Tea (with caffeine)

- Dinner
    - o   3 ounces of any type of meat (same size as deck of cards)
    - o   1 cup of green beans or lettuce, tomatoes, spinach
    - o   1/2 banana or 2 kiwis, 1 cup of papaya or 2 apricots
    - o   1 small apple – high in pectin, which limits the amount of fat your cells can absorb.
    - o   1 cup of vanilla ice cream – source of calcium – the more calcium is stored in fat cells, the more fat the cells will burn.

DAY 2:

- Breakfast
    - o   1 egg or a cup of milk or 2 slices of bacon
    - o   1 slice of toast (whole wheat)
    - o   1/2 banana

- Lunch
    - o   1 cup of cottage cheese or plain Greek yoghurt
    - o   1 hardboiled egg
    - o   5 saltine crackers or rice crackers

- Dinner
    - o   2 hot dogs (without bun) or cup of lentils
    - o   1 cup of broccoli or cauliflower
    - o   1/2 cup of carrots or celery or squash
    - o   1/2 banana
    - o   1/2 cup of vanilla ice cream or 1 cup of fruit flavored yogurt or apple juice

DAY 3:

- Breakfast
    - o   5 saltine crackers or any gluten free cracker
    - o   1 slice of cheddar cheese or soy cheese or tofu
    - o   1 small apple or dried apricots or plums and peaches
- Lunch
    - o   1 hardboiled egg (or cooked however you like)
    - o   1 slice of toast (whole wheat)
- Dinner
    - o   1 cup of tuna
    - o   1/2 banana or plums, grapes and apple
    - o   1 cup of vanilla ice cream

And for the **non-fasting days**, here are some suggestions for the 1500 calorie hours:

Breakfast (Choose ONE of the following per day):

- Yogurt Parfait: 1 cup of plain yogurt layered with 1 cup mixed berries, 1/4 cup granola and 1 tablespoon of sliced almonds.
- Cheerful morning: 1 cup milk, 1 sliced banana and 1 cup cheerios. You can also eat 1 orange.
- Egg on toast: 1 egg scrambled in 1 teaspoon butter on a slice of whole grain toast with tomato slices and 1/4 avocado sliced.
- Bagel and lox: 1/2 whole-wheat bagel topped with 1 tablespoon cream cheese and 1 oz smoked salmon. Add thin tomato, cucumber and red onion slices.
- Cinnamon Oatmeal: 1/3 cup rolled oats cooked with 2/3 cup milk and 1/2 cup chopped apple. Top with 2 tablespoons of chopped walnuts & cinnamon.
- Walnut Waffles and Berries: 2 whole grain waffles topped with 1/4 cup strawberries and 1/4 blueberries and 7 walnuts.
- Florentine Egg and English Muffin: scramble 2 eggs and 1 cup fresh spinach and eat on top of a whole wheat toasted English muffin.

- Pear and Almond-Butter Toast: one slice of whole wheat toast topped with 1 tablespoon almond butter and 1 pear sliced.

- Tomato-Basil Ricotta Toast: one slice of whole wheat toast topped with 1/3 cup ricotta cheese, 4 slices of tomato and fresh basil leaves.

- Banana & Honey Smoothie: Blend (in a blender) 1 cup plain soy milk, 1 banana, 1 tablespoon honey, 2 tablespoons oatmeal and 1 tablespoon of flax seeds.

- Cheesy Omelet: 2 egg omelette with cheddar cheese.

- Protein intake: 2 lean sausages, 1 soft boiled egg and a kiwi fruit

Lunch (Choose ONE of the following per day):

- Tuna Pita: Mix 1/2 can of tuna with 1/4 cup white beans, 1 teaspoon of olive oil and 1 teaspoon of lemon juice. Serve in a 4-inch whole-wheat pita with 2 leaves lettuce. Eat 1 cup of grapes on the side.

- Protein Salad: Toss 2 cups lettuce, 1 cup chopped raw vegetables, 1 hard-boiled egg, 2 teaspoons of raisins and 2 teaspoons of almonds. Top with 2 teaspoons of balsamic dressing.

- Mediterranean Plate: 1 piece of whole-wheat pita bread stuffed with 1-ounce feta cheese, 1 cup of tomatoes, 6 olives, 1/4 cup hummus and 1 cup raw spinach drizzled with 1 teaspoon of olive oil and 1 teaspoon of lemon juice.

- Veggie Lunch: 1 cup of lentil soup with 1 slice of toasted whole wheat bread topped with 1 teaspoon pesto, 2 tablespoons shredded mozzarella and 1 tablespoon chopped sun-dried tomatoes.

- Vegetarian Quesadilla: 1 whole-wheat tortilla stuffed with 1/3 cup shredded Cheddar, 1/4 cup black beans, 1/4 cup each sliced peppers & mushrooms, sautéed in 1 teaspoon olive oil. Serve with 1/4 avocado, sliced.

- Salad on the Military Diet - Tuna Walnut Greens: Toss 2 cups of spring greens, 3 ounces of tuna, 3 tablespoons of walnuts, and 1 cup of grape tomatoes cut in half. Top with 2 teaspoons of balsamic vinaigrette dressing.

- Turkey, Pear and Swiss Sandwich: 2 slices of whole grain bread with 1 teaspoon Dijon mustard, 5 slices of turkey, 1 pear sliced, and 1 slice of Swiss cheese.

- Black-Bean Wrap: Wrap 3/4 cup of black beans, 1/4 avocado, 1 cup of romaine lettuce, 2 tablespoons of salsa inside 2 whole wheat tortillas.

- Chicken Salad Pita: Mix together 1 cup diced and cooked chicken, 2 tablespoons balsamic vinegar, 1/4 cup chopped scallions, 1 stalk of chopped celery and 1 cup of salad greens. Stuff inside a whole wheat pita.

Dinner (Choose ONE of the following per day):

- BBQ Black Bean Burger and Slaw: 1 black bean burger cooked with 1 tablespoon BBQ sauce, served in a whole wheat bun. You can eat the slaw in the burger or on the side. Mix 1.5 cups of shredded cabbage, broccoli, cauliflower and carrots with 1 tablespoon apple cider vinegar with 2 tablespoons of olive oil.

- Shrimp and Zucchini Pasta: Cook 2 ounces frozen or fresh shrimp with 1 clove of garlic, 1 cup chopped zucchini, 2 tablespoons chopped fresh basil and 1 tablespoon of olive oil. Serve on one cup of whole wheat pasta noodles of your choice.

- Hot Peanut Chicken Wraps: Saute 2/3 cup of sliced chicken, 1/4 cup scallions, 2 tablespoons of peanuts, 1 tablespoon hot sauce and 1 cup of shredded cabbage, broccoli, cauliflower and carrot mix in cooking spray. Wrap all this in 2 whole wheat tortillas.

- Sushi: 1 cup miso soup, 1 Tuna roll and a small seaweed salad.

- Pepper Cilantro Fajitas: Cook 1 cup bell peppers (red, green or orange), 1/2 small onion and 1 tablespoon olive oil. Spread 1/2 cup refried beans on 2 whole wheat tortillas. Top with sautéed vegetables and cilantro.

- Black Bean and Zucchini Quesadilla: Sauté 1 cup chopped zucchini, 1/2 cup black beans, 2 teaspoons olive oil and 1 teaspoon of cumin. Place mixture on 2 whole wheat tortillas, sprinkle with 1/4 cup shredded cheddar. Fold in half and cook in a pan until the cheddar melts. Top with 2 teaspoons of salsa.

- Tortilla and Cheese Chili: 1.5 cups of warm vegetarian chili topped with 2 tablespoons of chopped scallions, 8 broken tortilla chips, 2 tablespoons shredded cheddar. Eat with a side salad: 2 cups mixed greens and 1 tablespoon Italian salad dressing.

- Florentine Goat Cheese Flatbread: Sauté 4 ounces of chicken, 3 cups of baby spinach, 2 teaspoons of olive oil, and 1 garlic clove. Put all this on a piece of whole grain flatbread, topped with 1-ounce goat cheese. Bake at 350 degrees for 5 minutes or so.

- Shrimp Fried Brown Rice: Sauté 1 cup cooked brown rice, 1 tablespoon sesame oil, 1 tablespoon soy sauce, 1 garlic clove and 1 tablespoon grated ginger. Then add 3 ounces of precooked shrimp and 2 cups of bok choy. Sauté another few minutes.

- Cheese and Artichoke Pizza with side salad: Top a whole grain flatbread with 3 tablespoons spaghetti sauce, 1/2 cup canned artichoke hearts, 2 tablespoons parmesan cheese, 1/4 cup mozzarella and bake for about 10 minutes. The side salad is 3 cups mixed greens, 2 tablespoons pine nuts and 2 tablespoons of Italian salad dressing.

- Stuffed Chili and Cheese Potato: Top a baked potato with 1/2 cup of turkey or vegetarian chili, 1 cup cooked broccoli and 1/4 cup shredded cheddar.

- Italian Sausage Pasta: Sauté 1 sliced Italian sausage, 1 garlic clove, 1/2 cup chopped mushrooms, 1/2 cup chopped onions and 1/2 cup chopped zucchini. Add in 1/2 cup spaghetti sauce to warm and serve over 3/4 cup of whole wheat pasta topped with 1 tablespoon grated parmesan cheese.

- Cajun Chicken with Rice: Sprinkle 1 teaspoon dried Cajun seasoning on 4 ounces of chicken breast. Bake or grill. Sauté 1 clove of garlic, 1/2 cup chopped onion, 1 bell pepper, in 2 teaspoons of olive oil. Add 2 tablespoons of tomato paste and a few sprinkles of Tabasco sauce. Add 3/4 cup of precooked brown rice. Serve the chicken on top of the rice.

Snacks (Choose **TWO** of the following per day):

- Fruit-and-nut bar
- 1 cup snap peas with 1/4 cup hummus
- 1 cup of cantaloupe with 1/2 cottage cheese
- 1 cup carrot sticks with 3 tablespoons of hummus
- 1 apple and 22 pistachios
- 12-oz latte and 1 clementine or mandarin orange
- 10 tortilla chips with 1/4 cup guacamole
- 1 banana with 1 tablespoon of peanut butter

- 2 Crispy rye crackers with 2 tablespoons of cream cheese
- 1 cup plain yogurt with 1 cup mixed berries
- 1/2 ounce raisins and 2 tablespoons soy nuts 14 almonds and an apple
- 1/2 cup sorbet 1-ounce chocolate-covered almonds
- 100-calorie mini bag popcorn
- 1-ounce string cheese and 4 whole-grain crackers
- 3 cups air popped popcorn, nothing added

LEAN GAINS

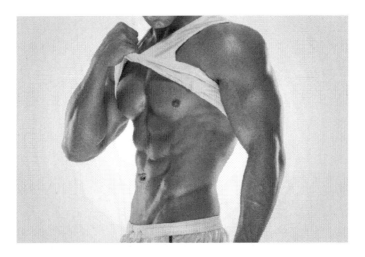

Calories: Use the *Harris-Benedict equation* to work out your personal optimum calorie intake. Remember, this plan is about ensuring that you have 16 hours without food every day.

Macronutrients: As this plan is focused on fasting as you work out, protein and fats are of highest priority, with carbohydrates being needed for energy to exercise.

The following plan is suggested for the LeanGains diet (these foods are all to be eaten within an 8-hour window, whether it's a rest day or a workout day):

Rest Day:

- 7 sticks lean pepperoni (840 cal, 98 pro, 21 carb, 56 fat)
- 700g egg whites (364 cal, 76 pro, 5 carb, 1 fat)
- 1 can tuna (90 cal, 20 pro, 0 carb, 1 fat)
- 10 liver tabs (80 cal, 20 pro, 0 carb, 0 fat)
- 680g soy milk (160 cal, 16 pro, 8 carb, 8 fat)
- 40g Hershey cocoa (80 cal, 8 pro, 24 carb, 4 fat)
- 900g zucchini (154 cal, 11 pro, 30 carb, 3 fat)
- TOTAL: 1768 Cal, 249 Pro, 88 Carb, 74 Fat

Workout Day:

- 1,890g soy milk (450 cal, 45 pro, 23 carb, 23 fat)

- 1 box kashi golean (980 cal, 91 pro, 140 carb, 7 fat)

- 1,500g Greek yogurt (857 cal, 154 pro, 51 carb, 0 fat)

- 600g blueberries (290 cal, 3 pro, 60 carb, 4 fat)

- 10x liver tabs (80 cal, 20 pro, 0 carb, 0 fat)

- 11g coconut oil (99 cal, 0 pro, 0 carb, 11 fat)

- TOTAL: 2756 Cal, 313 Pro, 274 Carb (not counting fiber), 45 Fat

This is a good example of the sorts of things you can be eating – the best way to get everything you need, whilst also working out to build up muscle. Try the LeanGains website *(leangains.com/2010/07/leangains-meals.html)* for lots of other meal ideas.

EAT STOP EAT

It is recommended for you to include a few fasting days in your week, every week. To do this, here is a sample 3-day plan, including fasting and non-fasting days to show how you should set up your own plan.

Calories: No calories on fasting days – water only. 1,500 to 2,500 calories (depending on your personalized situation and end goal) for the non-fasting days.

Macronutrients: The pyramid below shows all that you need to include in your Eat Stop Eat diet, and the quantities in which you need to consider them:

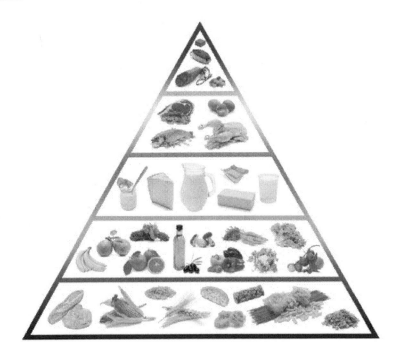

DAY 1:

- Breakfast – oatmeal, egg white omelet with olive oil, and an orange
- Mid-Morning – Greek yogurt with fresh blueberries
- Lunch – Chicken breast with spinach salad and olive oil dressing along with an apple
- Mid-Afternoon – Whey protein shake with a banana

- Dinner (at 5 pm) – Lean steak, baked sweet potato, steamed green beans with olive oil

- Begin FAST at 6pm

DAY 2:

- Continue FAST until 6 pm

- Dinner (at 6 pm) – Salmon with rice and two cups steamed broccoli

- Before Bed Snack – Cottage cheese with natural peanut butter

DAY 3:

- Breakfast – Toast with natural peanut butter and an egg white omelet

- Mid-Morning – Two hard boiled eggs with raw veggies

- Lunch – One can of tuna with spinach leaves, diced vegetables, and Italian salad dressing

- Mid-Afternoon – Greek yogurt with fresh strawberries

- Dinner – Grilled chicken with steamed Brussels sprouts drizzled with olive oil and lemon juice

- Before Bed – Cottage cheese with flaxseeds

As you can see, getting all of the right macronutrients is essential for this plan – and that's because you want your metabolism to be moving as quickly as possible.

THE WARRIOR DIET

This diet is all about consuming one large meal per day, under eating the rest of the time. It takes a lot of ideas from the Paleo Diet – which is all about eating what our ancestors ate. It goes by the theory *'if you couldn't find it 2,000 years ago, you shouldn't eat it now'*. With this plan, nothing is processed. All is raw, natural and extremely healthy.

Below is an example plan to assist you with fat burning.

Calories: You will want to calculate your ideal calorie consumption using the *Harris-Benedict equation*, then consider the majority of this amount for one meal.

Macronutrients: Protein is important during the fasting period, carbohydrates and fats during the non-fasting time.

Breakfast:

- 5g BCAA (optional but helpful)
- 6oz 0% fat Greek Yogurt
- 3g fish oil

Lunch:

- 5g BCAA (optional)
- 1 scoop low carbohydrates protein powder or 2oz lean meat
- 1oz raw almonds

Pre Workout:

- 5g BCAA (optional)
- 1 scoop low carbohydrates protein powder
- 1 slice Ezekiel bread

During Workout:

- 1 scoop low carbohydrates protein powder

Post Workout:

- 1 scoop low carbohydrates protein powder
- 50g Swedish Oat starch/Waxy maize/Maltose/Dextrose/8oz sweet potato

Dinner:

- 14oz cooked chicken breast or 14oz top round steak
- 2 scoops casein based protein powder
- 3g Fish Oil
- 1 Food for Life Brown Rice bread English muffin drizzled with 1tbsp honey
- 8oz cooked sweet potato
- 2tbsp natural peanut butter
- 1tbsp coconut oil

Totals: 2340 Calories, 270g protein, 180g carbs, 45g fat.

This meal is very important, so it's best to make it yourself so you know exactly what has gone into it. It's also a good idea to eat mindfully, chewing slowly and taking notice of every bite, to get the maximum pleasure and benefit out of your meal.

FAT LOSS FOREVER

Fat Loss Forever, the diet that is tailed exactly to your personal needs, gives a sample diet for you to look at.

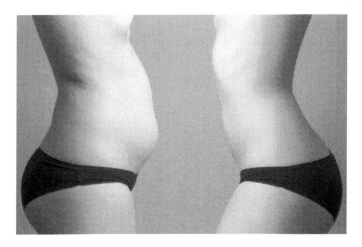

Here is some of the information from this sample diet:

Calories: This will be tailored to you. It's likely to be between 0 – 500 on fasting days, and 1500 – 2500 on non-fasting days.

Macronutrients: This will depend on your personalized needs from your plan. It's likely to include higher quantities of protein.

As stated previously, this diet recommends consuming this amount per day for one of their plans:

- Vegetables – 1 serving, 2 times a day
- Fruits – 1 serving, 2 times a day
- 100gm lean meat, 2 times a day
- 2 Thin Sunrice Rice Cakes or 2 melba toasts or 2 grissini breadsticks – daily
- The juice of one lemon each day (optional)
- Fresh herbs and spices– unlimited

You could select food from the following lists:

NB: If the food is not listed then it is NOT ALLOWED

Group 1	Protein: 2 serves per day	Raw Weight **100gms per serve** Weigh precisely – do not guess. – total protein per day is 200gms	White fish (no salmon, tuna etc.) Prawns Crab Crayfish Chicken breast Turkey Breast Lean Beef Veal PPX Pea Powder Shake Vegetarians: 1 egg + 2 egg whites Tofu Quorn PPX PeaPowder Shake
Group 2	Vegetables: 2 serves per day	Fresh or Frozen: Choose 1 vegetable per serve 2 serves per day only to be consumed with your protein serve 1 serve = approx. 2 cups *Exceptions to quantity*: Baby spinach raw 7 Cups Lettuce 6 cups Bok choy 5 cups	Asparagus Broccoli Cabbage Capsicum Cauliflower Spinach Lettuce Cucumber Tomato Fennel Zucchini Mushrooms

Group 3	Fruit: 2 serves per day + One fresh lemon for juice if desired	No Canned or dried fruits: Only Fresh	Apple Or Orange Or A handful of Strawberries Or ½ Grapefruit
Group 4	Bread/Grains: 2 serves per day	Each Serve is 1 slice	Choose from: Melba Toast Or Thin Rice Cake (plain) Or Grissino
Group 5	Condiments In Moderation	No butter, fats, oils, grease or bottled sauces. No stock cubes, vegemite, sugar etc.	Only choose from: Salt & pepper Herb & Spices: Coriander Parsley, thyme, basil, curry powder, chilies, ginger, cinnamon etc.
Group 6	Liquids: 3 or more litres water per day NO ALCOHOL 1 tablespoon of milk is allowed per day.	Plain Water/mineral water/soda water lots (9 – 20 glasses per day) No sweeteners/sugar: Use Stevia or Xylitol	You can also choose: Black tea, Black Coffee Chinese or Jasmine Tea

This *is* a plan that you'll have to pay for. However, the advice you get will be just for you, so will help you see guaranteed results.

UpDayDownDay DIET

For this diet plan, you fast and eat 'normally' on alternate days. You'll eat 500 – 600 calories on fasting days and 2000 – 2500 calories on non-fasting days. Here is a fast sample on what you could eat during your alternate fasting and non-fasting days.

Calories: 500 – 600 or 2000 (women) – 2500 (men) depending on the day.

Macronutrients: On the fasting days, ensure that you mostly eat proteins.

Here's how a **typical fasting day** would look like.

- Breakfast – 1 slice wholegrain toast with 1tbsp peanut butter

- Lunch – Bowl of Asian chicken noodle soup made from chicken broth, courgette, peppers, spring onions, a little cooked chicken breast, a small amount of noodles and hot pepper sauce.

- Dinner – Turkey chili made from a little minced turkey, garlic, pepper, chili, canned tomatoes, white beans e.g. cannellini, spices and herbs.

Total: 529 calories.

And here is a sample **non-fasting day** of full calories. You *can* eat as normal on these days, or you can select to follow a healthier eating plan, such as this one:

Breakfast:

- Egg Muffin (1 egg, 1/2-ounce ham, 1 slice low-fat cheese, 1 English muffin, 1 tsp. reduced-fat margarine)

- Orange Juice (1 cup)

Morning Snack:

- Fruit Yogurt (1 cup) & Bran Mix (1 T.)

- Water with Lime Twist (1 cup)

Lunch:

- Tropical Chicken Salad (1.5-ounce chicken breast, 1/8 cup low-fat cottage cheese, 1.5 ounces' pineapple, 1 teaspoon reduced-calorie mayonnaise, orange peel, 1/4 cup grapes, 1/8 cup water chestnuts, chives, 1/8 cup tangerines, 1 cup spinach, 1 tsp. almonds)

- Three Bean Salad (1/3 cup each green beans, yellow beans and kidney beans; onion, vinegar, sugar substitute)

- Reduced-Fat Wheat Crackers (4 crackers)

- Baked Apple (1/2 large)

- Iced Tea with Lemon (1 cup)

Afternoon Snack:

- Fat-Free Fig Bars (2 bars)

- Skim Milk (1 cup)

Dinner:

- Garlic Chicken (5 ounces cooked chicken breast, 1/4 cup light wheat bread crumbs, 1/8 cup skim milk, 1/4 garlic clove, 1 tsp. tabasco, lemon juice)

- Wild Rice (1 cup)

- Zucchini/Summer Squash Medley (1 cup)

- Light Pound Cake (1 serving, topped with strawberries (1/4 cup) and whipped topping (2 T).

- Diet Soda (12 ounces)

Daily Totals:

- 1929 calories

- 250 grams carbohydrate

- 140 grams protein

- 41 grams fat

- 12 grams saturated fat

This is one of the most popular diet plans because it's quite easy to stick to. The fact that you only fast every other day, makes it seem much less of a diet and much more of a simple lifestyle change. If you use your 500 calories well, it can barely feel like you're dieting at all. Just be careful not to go over the top on the non-fasting days. If you binge eat, then you'll undo all of your hard work and end up feeling sluggish. The better you eat on the non-fasting days, the easier the fasting days will feel.

5:2 DIET

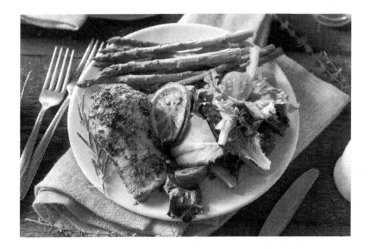

This diet is for two out of seven days a week. You will eat 500 – 600 days on two days, the other days you'll consume 2000 – 2500 calories. These days don't have to be fixed, you can change them to suit whatever you have going on, making this diet perfect if you have a chaotic, busy lifestyle. The following diet plan for this fast is suggested:

Calories: 500 – 600 for two days a week, 2000 – 2500 for the non-fasting days.

Macronutrients: Ensure that you get a balanced mix of proteins, fats and carbohydrates on the non-fasting days, but concentrate on protein for energy on the fasting days.

5 Options for the Non-Fast Days:

Breakfast:

- Medium bowl of porridge with 1 tablespoon of blanched almonds, 1 tsp of sunflower seeds made with water, sweetened with 5 drops of vanilla essence and 1 grated apple. Enjoy with one cup of green tea.

- 200g of Greek style full fat yoghurt with 100g of mixed berries (may be taken from frozen), 2 tsp of pumpkin seeds.

- 2 full egg omelet with large handful of wilted watercress or spinach, 1 piece of pumpernickel toast. 1 cup of white tea.

- Crumbled feta with half an avocado and lime juice on toasted rye. 1 cup of green tea.

- 2 slices of honey roast ham with two poached eggs. 1 cup of Rooibosch tea.

Lunch:

- Medium box of mixed fish sushi with small pot of edamame beans and optional bowl of miso soup

- Poached salmon with small potato salad and mixed leaf bag salad, served with olive oil and lemon juice dressing

- Chicken Caesar salad with added small pack of sugar snap peas, 1 dessert spoon of olive oil (instead of any pre-made dressing)

- Mixed bean hot pot with added soba noodles (buckwheat)

- 450g of fresh chicken and vegetable soup (not tinned), with two rye crackers

Dinner:

- 6oz fillet steak with potato dauphinoise and French beans

- Grilled sea bass (whole) with roasted root vegetables

- Tofu and Asian vegetables stir fry with soya, ginger and garlic sauce

- Lentil and vegetable bake with crumbled feta topping

- Fish pie with salmon, haddock and prawns

2 Options for the Fast Days:

Breakfast:

- 1 banana, 1 tsp of vanilla essence, 100g Greek style natural yoghurt (not low fat) - blend until smooth (add a dash of semi-skimmed milk for desired consistency)

- 2 poached eggs on a handful of wilted spinach

Lunch or Dinner:

- Small grilled chicken breast (skin removed) with 100g tabouleh salad

- 3 medium falafel grilled with 2 dessertspoon tahini dressing with a cucumber and tomato salad

Drinks Options – **Aim to drink 2 liters of fluids per day.**

- Herbal Teas – green, white, nettle, fennel, rooibosch, vanilla, jasmine, chamomile, ginger and lemon, peppermint

- Still water

- Sparkling water with Ginger juice extract, juice of two limes with 3 drops of vanilla essence and Lemongrass (1 stick, smashed not sliced).

This fast is a great way to eat a balanced, healthy diet, while losing weight. If you do it right and eat a lot of raw, fresh food, you'll feel much more energized, switched on and you'll also find it easier to ward off infections.

SPONTANEOUS MEAL SKIPPING

With this plan, you can choose what meal you want to skip. Some people prefer to avoid breakfast, some people are too busy to eat lunch and some people prefer to leave food out in the evening. Here is an example of requirements for your 2 daily meals.

Calories: You need to aim for 1500 – 2000 calories per day, although the beauty of this plan is that it *is* flexible so you don't have to be too strict about what you're eating. Skip meals according to what feels right for you.

Macronutrients: If skipping a meal, it's important to ensure that you're getting the right mix of proteins, fats and carbohydrates.

To achieve this goal, you could have half of your calories consumed around midday and then consume the second portion of your calories for a day in a big dinner.

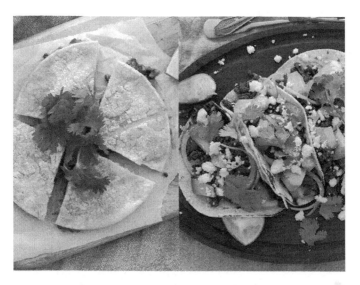

You can eat what you want on this plan, as long as you skip meals when you aren't hungry. As previously stated, this diet is all about getting in tune with your body, and learning exactly what it wants, and giving it that. You'll start to see how much more energy you get when you're only eating when necessary. This will lead to you feeling much healthier overall.

NATURAL NIGHTLY FASTING

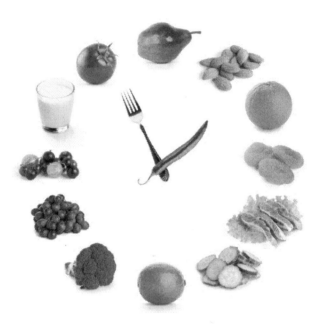

When you nightly fast, you continue to eat as normal, but leave at least 10 hours' food free – including the hours when you're sleeping. This leaves the evenings food free, helping you to lose weight and feel better.

Calories: Use the *Harris-Benedict equation* to find a more personalized recommendation of how many calories you should consume during your non fasting hours. This is likely to range between 1500 and 2500 calories per day.

Macronutrients: If you struggle with the fasting period, then it's best to eat your proteins and fats early in the day, and save your carbohydrates for later on.

Here's what you need to include on your plate for a balanced diet. When you divide these things up into manageable meals, they can look something like this:

- Breakfast – 2 ounces of grains, 1 cup of dairy and 1/2 cup of fruit.

- Lunch – 1 cup of vegetables, 1/2 cup of fruit, 2 ounces of grains, 1 cup of dairy and 2 ounces of protein.

- Dinner – 1 cup of vegetables, 1 cup of fruit, 2 ounces of grains, 1 cup of dairy and 3 1/2 ounces of protein for dinner.

Below are some examples of good meals you could be eating during the week throughout non-fasting hours:

Monday:

- Breakfast: Omelet with various vegetables, fried in butter or coconut oil.
- Lunch: Grass-fed yogurt with blueberries and a handful of almonds.
- Dinner: Cheeseburger (no bun), served with vegetables and salsa sauce.

Tuesday:

- Breakfast: Bacon and eggs.
- Lunch: Leftover burgers and veggies from the night before.
- Dinner: Salmon with butter and vegetables.

Wednesday:

- Breakfast: Eggs and vegetables, fried in butter or coconut oil.
- Lunch: Shrimp salad with some olive oil.
- Dinner: Grilled chicken with vegetables.

Thursday:

- Breakfast: Omelet with various vegetables, fried in butter or coconut oil.
- Lunch: Smoothie with coconut milk, berries, almonds and protein powder.
- Dinner: Steak and veggies.

Friday:

- Breakfast: Bacon and Eggs.
- Lunch: Chicken salad with some olive oil.

- Dinner: Pork chops with vegetables.

Saturday:

- Breakfast: Omelet with various veggies.
- Lunch: Grass-fed yogurt with berries, coconut flakes and a handful of walnuts.
- Dinner: Meatballs with vegetables.

Sunday:

- Breakfast: Bacon and Eggs.
- Lunch: Smoothie with coconut milk, a bit of heavy cream, chocolate-flavored protein powder and berries.
- Dinner: Grilled chicken wings with some raw spinach on the side.

We've all heard that eating late at night is bad for us and causes us to keep weight on, so if weight loss is your end goal with fasting then this is a great one to try.

CARB BACKLOADING

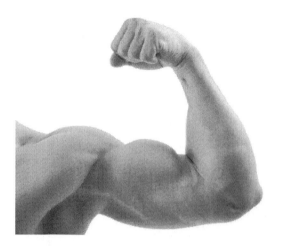

This plan is all about working out and fasting at the same time. If you want to build up muscle and gain the body that your desire, while gaining the health benefits that come with fasting, then this is the diet you should try. Below is suggested menu for you to try:

Calories: You will need to use the *Harris-Benedict equation* to work out how many calories you'll need to eat in a day, because the amount you exercise really comes into play with this diet.

Macronutrients: Of course this diet is mainly focused on carbohydrates, but don't forget to include proteins and fats too.

- *Breakfast:* Mushroom and spinach omelet provides filling fiber and essential amino acids.

- *Lunch:* Tuna salad with avocado and black olives is packed with protein to build muscles and unsaturated fats to keep your heart healthy.

- *Dinner:* Paella (1tbsp olive oil, 2 chicken breasts, 4 – 6 chicken wings, 2 cloves garlic, crushed, 1 red pepper, sliced, 1/2 tsp smoked paprika, 300g paella rice, 200g chorizo, 1-liter chicken stock, 8 cherry tomatoes, halved, pinch of saffron, 400g can cannellini beans, 50g frozen peas, 12 prawns, 12 mussels – serves 3 – 4).

    o Warm the oil in a frying pan over a medium heat.

    o Add the chicken and fry, turning occasionally, until it's slightly browned on all sides.

- o Add the garlic, peppers, paprika and rice and fry for two to three minutes.
- o Add the chorizo, stock, cherry tomatoes and saffron and cook for ten minutes.
- o Add the cannellini beans and peas and cook for another ten minutes.
- o Add the seafood and cook for a further ten minutes. If the liquid fully reduces, top up with boiling water to ensure the paella doesn't dry out and stick.
- *Snacks:* Satsuma's and cashew nuts provide immunity-boosting vitamins A and C, plus a decent serving of muscle-repairing protein.

Here is another plan, which you could try (remember to leave an 8-hour window for fasting)

- Upon Waking:
  - o 10g whey isolate; 1 tbs coconut oil; 5g creatine, coffee
- Breakfast:
  - o 1 bell pepper
  - o 1 cup spinach
  - o 3 large eggs scrambled
  - o 1/2 avocado
  - o 1/4 cup of cheese
  - o 1 fish oil pill
  - o Snack (optional):
  - o 1/4 almonds
  - o 5 celery stalks
- Lunch:
  - o 6oz chicken
  - o 1 broccoli
  - o 1 tbsp. olive oil
  - o Snack (optional):
  - o 1/4 almonds
  - o 2 hardboiled eggs

- o Pre-Training:
- o 25g whey isolate; 2 tbs coconut oil
- o Post-Training:
- o some protein shake with lots of carbs
- Dinner:
  - o 4oz salmon
  - o 14oz potato
  - o 2 cups jasmine rice
  - o 1 tbsp. butter
  - o Splurge:
  - o 2 cups lactose free milk
  - o 4 cups frosted corn flakes
  - o Last meal before fasting:
  - o 1/2 cup 2% cottage cheese

This diet has been designed for people who work out a lot – bodybuilders, etc. Only undertake this plan if you do a lot of exercise, otherwise it may leave you feeling sluggish.

Of course these diet plans are merely samples to give you some ideas and get you started. The beauty of the fast is the ability to eat *what* you want at certain times.

4. Prepare yourself.

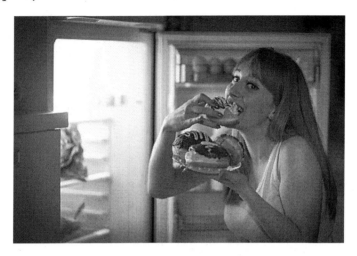

One of the hardest things about preparing yourself for a fast is getting over your **addiction to food**. This may be something that you don't even realize you have, which is why below is a list of signs to look out for:

- You end up eating more than planned when you start eating certain foods.

- You keep eating certain foods even if you're no longer hungry.

- You eat to the point of feeling ill.

- You worry about not eating certain types of foods or worry about cutting down on certain types of foods.

- When certain foods aren't available, you go out of your way to obtain them.

- You eat certain foods so often or in such large amounts that you start eating food instead of working, spending time with the family, or doing recreational activities.

- You avoid professional or social situations where certain foods are available because of fear of overeating.

- You have problems functioning effectively at your job or school because of food and eating.

If this is the case, you will need to *get some help from a health professional*. This addiction can be problematic and can get in the way of your dieting. It is generally associated with junk food, but can also relate to carbohydrates – this will also cause you issues with your fast. Below are **some tips for assisting you** with this:

- Look into the problem, not the symptom – often these addictions are related to something deeper than just food. Solving this can help you a lot.

- Phase out processed foods – this sort of food is unhealthy, and ridding yourself of it will only make you healthier.

- Be patient – of course this is going to be difficult, but you need to stick with it. The first 48 hours will be the hardest, but also the most rewarding.

- Break old habits – find out when you're eating badly and focus on that time.

- Slowly lower your intake – don't do it too fast because you'll have difficulties.

- Meet your nutritional needs – whatever you're doing, just be sure that you're getting everything you need.

- Have a cheat meal – don't deprive yourself or you'll find it harder to recover.

Another area where planning is going to be important while you fast is **exercise**. Your plan is going to change according to days where you're not eating, and being aware of this will help you in the long run.

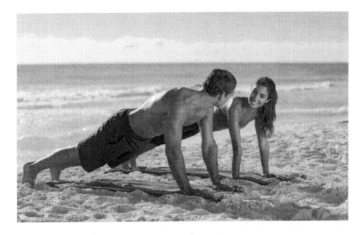

It is suggested that there are actually a lot of **benefits to exercising on an empty stomach** – if this is something that you'd wish to consider. These include:

- Decrease in body fat

- Improved muscle tone

- Improved athletic speed and performance

- Ability to achieve your fitness goals much faster

- Increase in energy and sexual desire

- Firmer skin and reduced wrinkles

It is actually recommended to do an **interval training** to get the most out of your workout. As long as you time your meals accordingly, you should have no issue with exercising during the days you fast. Here is an example of an easy workout you can do:

- Warm up for three minutes.

- Exercise as hard and fast as you can for 30 seconds. You should be gasping for breath and feel like you couldn't possibly go on another few seconds. It is better to use lower resistance and higher repetitions to increase your heart rate.

- Recover for 90 seconds, still moving, but at slower pace and decreased resistance.

- Repeat the high-intensity exercise and recovery 7 more times.

It's very important to remember that fasting isn't *only* for weight loss. It can also help you build up muscle mass – which has been demonstrated by the varying diets that have been included within this guide. Here are some **tips for exercising and building muscle as you fast:**

- Late night training sessions will help you manage when to eat.

- You need to consider protein and carbohydrates in your meal during the recovery period.

- Consume the bulk of your calories – about 60% – immediately after your workout, to assist your body in recovery.

- Eat about 20% of your daily calories before you workout to give you the energy that you'll need (while as stated above this is not actually necessary, but is should help in muscle mass building).

- Don't eliminate all fats – keep 'good' fats as a big part of your diet.

- Aim to eat before 5am – eating earlier rather than later is advised.

If you want to read more about building muscle and intermittent fasting, **Breaking Muscle** is a brilliant resource (*breakingmuscle.com/nutrition/build-lean-muscle-with-intermittent-fasting-carb-and-calorie-cycling*), filled with dieting and exercise tips.

If building muscle isn't your end goal, and the fasting is more about **burning fat,** you could also consider cardio exercises, such as running, swimming and sports, to combine with one of the fasting diets. It is really advisable to do at least *some* exercise alongside your fasting for the best results. Not only will you see your efforts working much quicker, you will also start to feel healthier and more energetic sooner. You are free to pick an exercise regime that suits you, as long as you do *something*.

Whatever the end goal, it's extremely important to consider **what you do after you work out.** This is your resting period, when your body recovers. This is the most important time for weight loss and muscle building, so establishing a great routine is essential for getting the most out of your exercise.

It is recommended that you do the following:

- *Cool Down* – do some sort of light cardio to allow your body to adjust and your heart rate to slow down. Five minutes is recommended.

- *Stretch* – after this, you should stretch. Your muscles have contracted and you don't want them to shrink. Doing this will allow your body to recover properly.

- *Drink Water* – replenish your fluid levels. Drink 2 to 3 cups during the 2 hours after you've finished working out.

- *Refuel* – eating is also important after working out. It helps you repair your muscles and boost your energy levels. This needs to be done within 90 minutes after you've finished working out. Include protein and carbohydrates in this meal or snack.

5. Things to remember.

There are things to keep in mind the entire time you're fasting, to keep you going. These include:

- **One day at a time** – don't worry too much about the future, just focus on where you are.

- **Goals** – that being said, always have your goals in mind, for motivation.

- **Caffeine** – this is great for the pick-me-ups you're going to need along the way.

- **Water** – keep hydrated at all times. This is very important.

- **Rewards** – always reward yourself for achieving goals. This will help keep you motivated. This doesn't have to be food rewards; you can think outside the box for it.

- **Sugar** – find other treats that don't involve sugar. You can retrain your brain to enjoy healthy snacks just as much. It just takes a little time.

- **Don't get caught up in the rules** – focusing too hard on the 'dos and don'ts' can actually be unhelpful.

- **Don't be too hard on yourself** – even if you make mistakes, it isn't the end of the world. You can always start again.

- **Don't gorge** – when you can finally eat again, don't go too mad. It'll make you feel awful and will undo a lot of your hard work.

- **Plan** – if you're dedicated to getting something from all of your food groups, your fast will likely be more successful. You may just need to plan your meals in advance.

6. Get started!

So now you are ready! Once you've covered all of these steps, there is nothing holding you back, so get started. No more excuses, no more holding back, just begin. There is no time like the present, the longer you put it off, the more chance you'll never begin. So don't think *'I'll start on Monday'*, *'I'll do it on the first of the month'* or *'I'll begin when so-and-so is over'*. Unless there is a genuine reason that is going to get in your way, just get going!

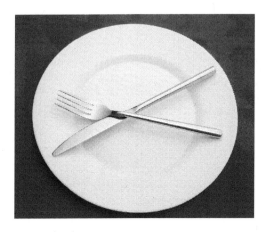

Here are the **practical steps to beginning** recapped:

- *Set your objective* – Chose your goal and keep it in mind throughout. Pick a fasting plan according to your aim and your lifestyle. It needs to be achievable to ensure that you stick to it. If it's simply impossible, it'll never happen!

- *Make your commitment* – Once you set your mind to the intermittent fast, ensure that you stick to it. Do whatever it takes to ensure that you won't go off track – even if this means telling someone and making sure they hold you accountable.

- *Plan and prepare* – Get everything in place. Make sure nothing will hold you back. Once the fasting has become a habit, ingrained in your everyday routine, this will become easier, but the first few days and weeks will be where the biggest challenge lies. Make sure that these are days where you can rest where necessary, but you have enough distraction to keep you going.

- *Shop* – Ensure that you have all the food you're going to need already in your cupboards. You don't want any excuse to give up. This also goes for workout equipment.

12 INTERMITTENT FASTING TRICKS TO MAKE IT WORK

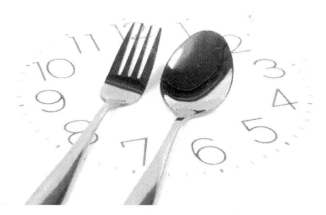

Here are some **tips and tricks for ensuring that you have a successful fast:**

1. Drink lots of water – men should aim for at least 3 to 4 liters per day, and women 1.5 to 2 liters. Be sure to have your first glass first thing in the morning.

2. Drink coffee and tea to keep your appetite at bay because caffeine is a natural suppressant.

3. Keep yourself busy and do meaningful work. The busier you are, the

less you'll be thinking about food. Get out of the house wherever possible!

4. Get your best most productive work done in the morning because you'll be the most motivated and have lots of energy.

5. Make it flexible for you – creating your own fast is the best way to really make it work, as if the fast fits around your lifestyle, you'll be more likely to stick to it. Play around with the diets until you find one that fits.

6. Give it a good go for at least 3 weeks – don't give up too quickly. It takes this amount of time for your body to adjust.

7. Use supplements to your advantage. Branched Chain Amino Acids can help you with anything missing from your diet.

8. Try delaying breakfast to see how long you can hold it off for. This can give you a good guideline for the best fasting and eating times for you.

9. Don't tell people you are fasting – the less people that know, the less 'helpful opinions' you'll be forced to hear. You are doing this for *you*. Don't forget that.

10. Don't forget to use exercise to your advantage. Workout with weights to help build your muscle, which in turn increases your metabolism.

11. Protein is your friend. Include it in every single meal if possible, and use supplements to help you out too.

12. Eat right. Don't use your non fasting days to eat rubbish. That will hinder you in the long run. It's important to remember that the first meal of the day will set the tone for the rest of the day. Make it a healthy one!

SAFETY MEASURES THAT YOU SHOULD KNOW

There are some factors that you will need to be aware of before starting your fast, and this chapter will cover them.

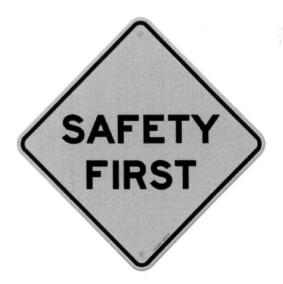

Side Effects

Here are some of the possible side effects that you might experience whilst fasting:

- Becoming obsessed with food – especially in the early weeks.

- Rationalizing overeating because you're fasting for a set amount of hours per day.

- Feeling overly full after eating.

- Lower energy levels – especially in the morning.

You may also feel:

- Hunger – particularly at first.

- You may feel weakness and like your brain isn't functioning properly.

- A dependence on caffeine for an energy boost.

Being aware of these factors will help you to cope with them if they come around. Sometimes just knowing that what you're going through is normal can be hugely beneficial.

Safety Measures

To confirm that intermittent fasting is safe for you, you'll need to speak to a health professional that can judge your personalized situation. However, here are a few tips to get you started.

For starters, there are **people that shouldn't fast**:

- *Pregnant and nursing women* – the effects on the baby and fetus are currently unknown.

- *Children* – in America it's frowned upon to let a child fast. However, in Europe, it's permissible under the care of a health professional if the child is obese and has made the decision on their own accord.

- *Those with certain medical conditions* – those who suffer from liver or kidney weakness or disease should avoid fasting. So should those who are extremely frail, malnourished, anemic, or exhausted. It's also advisable to consult a doctor if you have a weakened immune system, severely high blood pressure, diabetes, or weak circulation causing frequent fainting.

- *Those with eating disorders* – such as anorexia or bulimia.

- *After surgery or a major illness* – time should be taken to recuperate before attempting a fast. Also, don't fast directly prior to major surgery.

- *Anyone who is afraid of fasting* – fear does not put you in the proper frame of mind for fasting and can lead to an unpleasant experience. Strong emotions, such as fear, are known to alter the body's physiological processes. It can shut down certain bodily functions. It also is a closed emotional state. Instead, someone embarking on a fast should be relaxed and confident, and feeling open to the positive changes fasting creates.

Insider Tips For
Breaking A Fast

Knowing when to stop fasting is key to doing it safely. When you experience *'true hunger'* – which means you need to listen to your body and read the signs of when you're done.

The dictionary describes **hunger** as *"the painful sensation or state of weakness caused by need of food."* Some people become irritable, shaky, or disoriented if they are not fed at their usual mealtime. Others experience hunger as feeling lightheaded, empty, low, headachy, or hollow. At times a growling stomach prompts an eating episode. Some eat when they get depressed. Others lose their appetite when they get depressed. External stimuli are abundant, as are emotional and physical ones, yet few of these are hunger, just some other strain on your nervous system.

Other signs it's **time to end the fast** include:

- Sudden sickness or nausea.
- Diarrhea.
- Rapid increase or decrease in your heart rate.
- Excessive dehydration.
- Sudden excessive weakness.
- Your intuition is usually a great indicator. Often you will know when your time is up.

It is suggested that the **adjustment period for breaking a fast is around 4 days**. Consuming easy to digest foods during this time is vital to all your system to get used to its new routine.

Ideas for ***things you could eat*** include (start adding the new foods from toward the top of the list):

- fruit and vegetable juices
- raw fruits
- vegetable or bone broths
- yogurt (or other living, cultured milk products), unsweetened

- lettuces and spinach (can use plain yogurt as a dressing and top with fresh fruit)

- cooked vegetables and vegetable soups

- raw vegetables

- well-cooked grains and beans

- nuts and eggs

- milk products (non-cultured)

- meats and anything else

More **tips for breaking a fast successfully**:

- Pay attention to the way that your body reacts to these new foods (above). Any adverse reactions are there for a reason.

- Look out for feeling full. Once you reach this, stop eating.

- Start with small, frequent meals. Eat every 2 hours or so, while slowly progressing towards larger, more normal sized meals.

- Always chew your food well as this aids digestion.

- Eat carefully to add live enzymes and good bacteria into your body. Fresh, raw foods are a great way to achieve this.

COMMON MISTAKES TO AVOID

This chapter will cover the errors you'll want to avoid in order to have a successful fast. Being aware of these gives you a much better chance at overcoming them.

Intermittent Fasting Myths Debunked

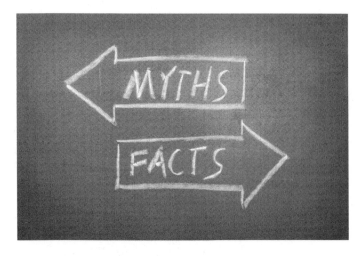

1. Skipping breakfast will make you fat.

The fact that there's something special about breakfast is a common misconception. The truth of this is more likely to lie in the fact that people who tend to skip breakfast are actually less health conscious overall. In fact, a scientific study (details of which can be found by going to the following link *ajcn.nutrition.org/content/early/2014/06/04/ajcn.114.089573.abstract*) conduct- ed in 2014 compared eating breakfast vs. skipping breakfast in 283 over- weight and obese adults. After a 16-week study period, there was no differ- ence in weight between groups.

2. Eating frequently boosts your metabolism.

While it's true that the body expends a certain amount of energy digesting and assimilating the nutrients in a meal, there's no difference in calories burned if you eat more frequently. Total calorie intake and macronutrient breakdown is what counts.

3. Eating frequently helps reduce hunger.

This depends on the individual. Many studies have been conducted and produced varying results. There is *no* evidence to suggest that snacking re- duces hunger for everyone.

4. Eating many smaller meals will help you lose weight.

Certain studies (e.g. *ncbi.nlm.nih.gov/pubmed/26024494*) have disproved this theory. For example, a study in 16 obese men and women did not find any difference in weight, fat loss or appetite when comparing 3 and 6 meals per day.

5. The brain needs a constant supply of glucose.

This theory is based on the presumption that the brain can only use glucose for fuel. However, this ignores the fact that the body can produce its own glucose from the supply left in the liver. Keytones can also be used if neces- sary.

6. Eating often is good for your health.

It's actually unnatural for the body to be constantly in a 'fed' state. In fact, studies (e.g. *ncbi.nlm.nih.gov/pmc/articles/PMC4265261*) show that where fast- ing can have positive effects on your health, eating too much can have a negative impact on your overall health.

7. Fasting puts your body in 'starvation mode'.

According to the claims, not eating makes your body think it is starving, so it shuts down its metabolism and prevents you from burning fat. It's actually true that long-term weight loss can reduce the amount of calories you burn. This is the true "starvation mode" (the technical term is *adaptive thermogenesis*).

However, this happens with weight loss no matter what method you use. There is no evidence that this happens more with intermittent fasting than other weight loss strategies.

8. The body can only use up a certain amount of protein per meal.

There are some who claim that we can only digest 30 grams of protein per meal, and that we should eat every 2-3 hours to maximize muscle gain. However, this is not supported by scientific studies.

The most important factor for most people is the total amount of protein consumed not how many meals it is spread over.

9. Intermittent fasting makes you lose muscle.

Some believe that we eventually start to burn muscle for fuel when fasting. In fact, calorie restriction doesn't have to work that way. Studies (e.g. *ncbi.nlm.nih.gov/pubmed/21410865*) prove that intermittent fasting is actually the best way to lose weight and maintain muscle.

10. Intermittent fasting is bad for your health.

As we've already seen from this book, there are actually a great number of health benefits that can be provided from completing an intermittent fast. The scientific evidence to support this claim is overwhelming.

11. Intermittent fasting makes you overeat.

Where it *is* possible to eat extra during your 'feeding window' to compensate for missing calories, it won't be a complete compensation. Scientific studies (e.g. *ncbi.nlm.nih.gov/pubmed/12461679*) show that on average, people who fasted for a whole day only ended up eating about 500 extra calories the next day.

So they expended about 2400 calories during the fasting day, then "overate" by 500 calories the day after. The total reduction in calorie intake was then 1900 calories, which is a very large deficit for only 2 days.

Why Are You Failing?

There are many reasons that you might be failing at fasting. You may have tried it numerous times, but have never quite managed to get it right. This doesn't mean that *you're* a failure, just that you may have been taking the wrong tactic for yourself.

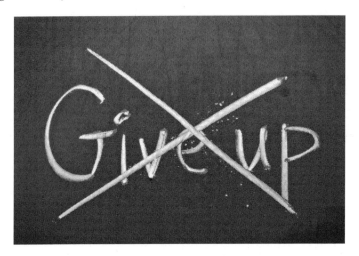

Look at **the common fasting pitfalls,** and how to avoid them:

- You may have picked a fast that doesn't suit you. Don't give up, simply learn from this and try again.

- Quitting at the first hurdle is bad news. There *will* be difficult times, but it will get easier if you continue to pursue.

- Don't smoke while fasting.

- Peer pressure from others can be challenging. Don't give in – this is for you not them.

- Avoid alcohol while you're completing the fast.

- Don't forget you goal. You're doing this for a reason, don't forget that.

- Illness can get in the way – that's unavoidable, don't use it as an excuse to give up.

- Life gets in the way. If this happens, don't be hard on yourself. Simply pick yourself up and start again.

- Remember that this *is* a lifestyle change. You will need to reconsider the way that you shop, the times you work out and the way you live your life. It'll all be worth it in the long run though!

- Do not resort to junk food – this is just empty calories that will do you harm in the long run.

10 PROVEN TIPS FOR MANAGING YOUR FAST

This chapter is going to cover the practical tips necessary for managing your fasting days. These will help you when you get started with your own intermittent fasting regime.

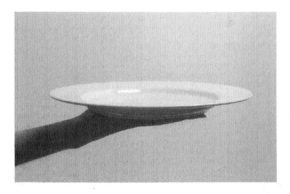

1. When you get hungry...

There are appetite suppressants that will help you get through the fasting window. These include water, caffeine, green tea, chia seeds and cinnamon. Use these to help you get through!

2. Combining fasting with exercise.

This *is* possible – in fact, many studies have shown that it's beneficial! After a while, you will work out what time of day is best for your workout. This was discussed in the previous chapter.

3. Getting dizzy or tired.

Generally, this is down to dehydration so ensure that you drink lots. It's also advisable to increase your salt intake – especially if headaches become an issue.

4. I'm already struggling!

The best way to prevent yourself from giving up is to keep busy. Take your mind off food by going out and doing something productive.

5. But I'm so busy.

This can work to your advantage as your mind won't always be on food. Before this becomes problematic, plan a fast that suits your current hours of work/commitments. There's no excuse not to do it – especially not this!

6. I keep gorging.

Once you have finished your fast, pretend it never happened and carry on as normal. This will get easier as time goes on and your body becomes adjusted.

7. Things keep cropping up.

This is why planning is essential. Clearing your schedule of anything important while you adjust will equate to how successful you are.

8. Meeting negativity.

Not everyone understands the benefits of fasting, which is why it's best to only tell those who need to know – family, close friends, etc. Others will try to put you off or psyche you out, preventing you from even beginning.

9. Maintaining the weight loss.

The fast isn't a quick fix. It's a long term lifestyle change which will help you maintain the slimmer/healthier figure that you want. To keep this up, it's also advisable to eat a lot healthier – all the time!

10. How to keep going.

If you feel tired, you need to rest. Your body is trying to tell you something and you need to listen. That is why it's advisable to clear your schedule in the beginning.

FAQ

1. What you can achieve with intermittent fasting?

One of the main things that you can achieve with intermittent fasting is a healthy weight loss. On top of this, you can also become much healthier, avoid certain diseases, and give yourself a lot more energy. The potential benefits that can come from an intermittent fast are endless.

2. Can you follow this plan if you have health issues? Is it suitable for people who have stomach problems such as ulcers, gastritis, and hyper acidity?

You can follow the intermittent fast no matter what, as long as you consult a health professional beforehand. Some experts believe that taking this stress off of your digestive system is actually good for stomach disorders. At **The Fast Diet** forum (*thefastdiet.co.uk/forums/topic/stomach-problems*), many people have described their stomach issues as improved due to fasting.

3. Is fasting suitable for everyone? Who should not do it?

Fasting is suitable for most people, but as described previously in this book, there *are* people who it isn't good for. These include pregnant women, children and those who suffer from certain illnesses. It's always advisable to consult your doctor before starting a fast – to get some personalized advice.

4. Is intermittent fasting safe?

Intermittent fasting is safe when performed correctly. Each diet shown in this book has been studied and undertaken by many people beforehand. However, speaking to a health professional can ensure that you chose the protocol that's right for you.

5. Is it difficult to take up?

Of course, there are challenges, which is why most people suggest that you give it a month before quitting – to give yourself adequate time to get used to the lifestyle change. You may experience tiredness, dizziness, dehydration, hunger, difficult emotions, etc. But, if you recognize these for what they are and pursue the plan anyway, you will end up with fantastic results.

6. What should you expect when you start fasting?

You can certainly expect some upheaval in your life as you adjust to this new plan. Yes, you might experience some of the negative side effects early on, but you can also expect an energy boost, adrenaline and a determination to carry on. Sticking with your fast will have wonderful results for you.

A study conducted by Precise Nutrition (*www.precisionnutrition.com*) picked up on the following comments from its participants:

"I learned that hunger is not an emergency."

"I learned that physical hunger is different from psychological hunger."

"I learned that eating is a privilege, some people in the world don't get to eat."

"I learned that eating is a responsibility, one that's to be taken seriously."

"I learned that food marketing is crazy. When fasting I notice food ads everywhere."

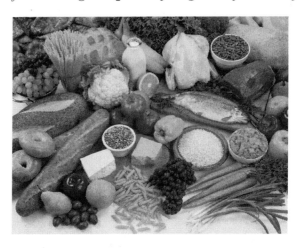

7. How long will results take to show?

The results will vary from person to person. Everyone is an individual and their body shape, metabolism and lifestyle is different – and this will impact on their results. On top of this, the diet you select and the dedication you give to it will also have an effect.

8. Will the fasting results be permanent? How do you maintain them?

Again, this will vary from person to person. Of course the results cannot be permanent if you end the fast and go on to gorge on junk food every day, but hopefully by the time you have decided to break you fast, you'll have a different attitude towards food. As you'll have noticed, the Fast Diet forum (*thefastdiet.co.uk/forums/topic/successful-maintenance-plans/*) is filled with ideas that other people have used to maintain their new bodies after fasting.

9. Can I combine different fasting methods?

It is possible to experiment with your fasting methods – adjusting them to suit you and your needs. Of course, it's always best to consult a doctor before doing this because you don't want to push things too far and make yourself ill.

10. How can intermittent fasting increase your energy?

Intermittent fasting increases your energy due to adrenaline and the use of keytones.

Fats are digested slowly and must be sent to the liver for processing (into ketones) before they can be used for energy. This process happens steadily and consistently, with no dramatic rises or falls in ketones (i.e. energy) available in the bloodstream.

The shorter, more-dramatic cycles of available energy during a fast that define carbohydrate metabolism are, quite simply, harder on the brain and metabolism. Intermittent fasting trains your body to switch to a more stable fuel source (fats) - and improvements in energy levels and cognitive performance come as a result.

11. If I'm a woman should I do anything differently?

The fasting rules for women are very similar to the fasting rules for men. The only difference might be the amount of calories you can consume during your 'feeding window'. The fasting protocols will cover this.

12. Can I fast without skipping breakfast?

The hours that you chose to perform the fast are entirely up to you. If you enjoy breakfast, then start your fast in the evening and throughout the night. Intermittent fasting is perfect for fitting around you.

13. Can you do the intermittent fast if pregnant or breastfeeding?

Pregnancy and breastfeeding is a very delicate time, which is why there aren't currently any fasting studies during this time. It is best to eat as normal during this period to ensure that your baby gets all the nutrients that it needs.

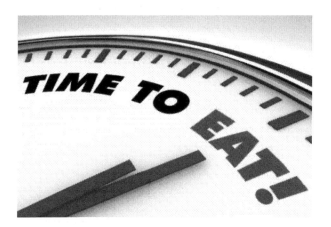

14. Is intermittent fasting safe for children?

Calorie restriction is frowned upon with children. There are cases when the doctor will allow it, so it's always best to consult with them before starting.

15. Can you intermittent fast if you're over 60?

This age group can be affected by the menopause. In this case, intermittent fasting can still be done, but the results may show themselves a lot slower. Again **The Fast Diet** forum (*thefastdiet.co.uk/forums/topic/fasting-weight-loss-and-menopause*) has some stories from some people who have experienced this.

16. Can you eat anything you like when you're fasting?

You *can* eat whatever you want during the 'feeding window', but it's advisable to save your calories for food that is worthwhile. Eating healthier, raw foods means that you can consume a lot more, and that more areas on the food pyramid will be covered. This will ensure that your body functions effectively.

17. How can intermittent fasting help with obesity?

Intermittent fasting has proven benefits for helping with weight loss, and this includes for people who suffer with obesity.

Many beliefs about obesity persist in the absence of supporting scientific evidence (presumptions); some persist despite contradicting evidence (myths). The promulgation of unsupported beliefs may yield poorly informed policy decisions, inaccurate clinical and public health recommendations, and an unproductive allocation of research resources and may divert attention away from useful, evidence-based information.

18. Are any vitamins or supplements necessary when fasting?

There are many supplements that can help you with your fast, discussed earlier in this book. Branched Chain Amino Acids is often considered one of the most important.

19. How do I find the perfect intermittent fast for me?

Finding the right fast for you might take some experimentation to see which style of fasting you prefer. It's also a good idea to work out your end goal before you start – there is no point in choosing the carb backloading plan if you wish to lose weight.

It's also a really sensible idea to see what is actually feasible for you to do. You'll need to consider your working hours, your exercise plan and your current upcoming plans, before making any decision. Speaking to a health professional beforehand is always advisable, so you can get some personalized advice.

20. Why shouldn't I eat 5 or 6 meals a day?

Once of the first problems with fasting, and consuming lots of smaller meals is that there isn't enough time in the non-fasting window to get them all in! However, it's also a bad idea on non-fasting day. Feeding this way will leave you eating all the time, which will actually leave you feeling *much* hungrier when you're not.

On top of this, eating this way is bad for your metabolism – it slows it down because it isn't given a break to work effectively. Your body also needs a rest for it to maintain muscle – so in all, it's much better to go for 2 or 3 meals instead.

21. How do I fit fasting into my busy lifestyle?

This is very simple – you need to select the fasting protocol that can work around you. If you can't find anywhere to fit in a three day fast, try natural nightly fasting instead. If you work random shifts, try the 5:2 diet – you can change the two fasting days week by week to suit you. Being busy is not an excuse not to give fasting a try – there are always ways that it can work.

22. How do I get started with intermittent fasting?

The steps to getting started with this sort of dieting can be found in the **Top Tips For Getting Started** chapter of this book. There you will find all of the advice that you need to get going with whichever fasting protocol you decide on.

Further advice can be found using the following resources:

James Clear at jamesclear.com/the-beginners-guide-to-intermittent-fasting

The IF Life at theiflife.com/intermittent-fasting-101-how-to-start-part-i/

Bodybuilding at bodybuilding.com/fun/to-eat-or-not-to-eat-your-fast-guide-to-fasting.html

These resources contain all sorts of advice, no matter what your end goal is. They will also take you on to further reading, ensuring that you can answer any questions that you have, and find out all that you need to know. The more knowledgeable you are, the more successful your fast will be.

CONCLUSION

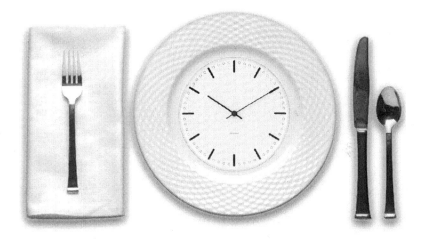

So as you have seen from all of the information included in this book, intermittent fasting can help your life tenfold. Just a few of the benefits provided by this diet include:

- It's scientifically proven to help you **lose weight** and stomach fat.

- It can **improve your health** – helping with conditions such as diabetes and heart issues.

- It can also help **ward off diseases**, helping you in the long run.

- It's really good for your brain.

- It can actually help you **live longer**.

There are many different diets that you can choose from and you can fit the fasting in with whatever time of day you're busy, to suit yourself. You can even keep exercising while you do the fast, so there really is no reason for you not to give it a go!

There *will* be times that you find it hard and there will be times that you want to give up, and that's the best time to seek advice from others, who have been through the same thing. Here are the links to some forums where you can connect with other fasters:

The Fast Diet at *thefastdiet.co.uk/forums/*

Fitness Through Fasting at *forum.fitnessthroughfasting.com*

Fast Day at *forum.fastday.com*

So good luck, and happy fasting!

ABOUT THE AUTHOR

Emily Moore has always had a passion for healthy living. It is what led her to study nutrition in university and to constantly be looking for new ways to help people live healthier lives. When she came across the idea of fasting, she was, at first, skeptical. But as she delved deeper and deeper into fasting and learned more and more about how intermittent fasting helps the body and solves many of the most common health problems in today's world, she began to realize the power that this lifestyle has and began working on a protocol to help bring this idea to the average person.

She has thoroughly studied fasting in all its forms, from water, to dry, to intermittent. She practices these types of diets in her own life and has worked with others to help them incorporate it into their lives. As she has done this, she watched people who have struggled with health issues all their lives become unburdened. She has seen the miracles that fasting can work on the people who do it correctly - that is why she wants to bring fasting to the masses, to help everyone solve their health problems, no matter what they are.

Printed in Great Britain
by Amazon